AUBREY DANCER

Meditation for the Easily Distracted

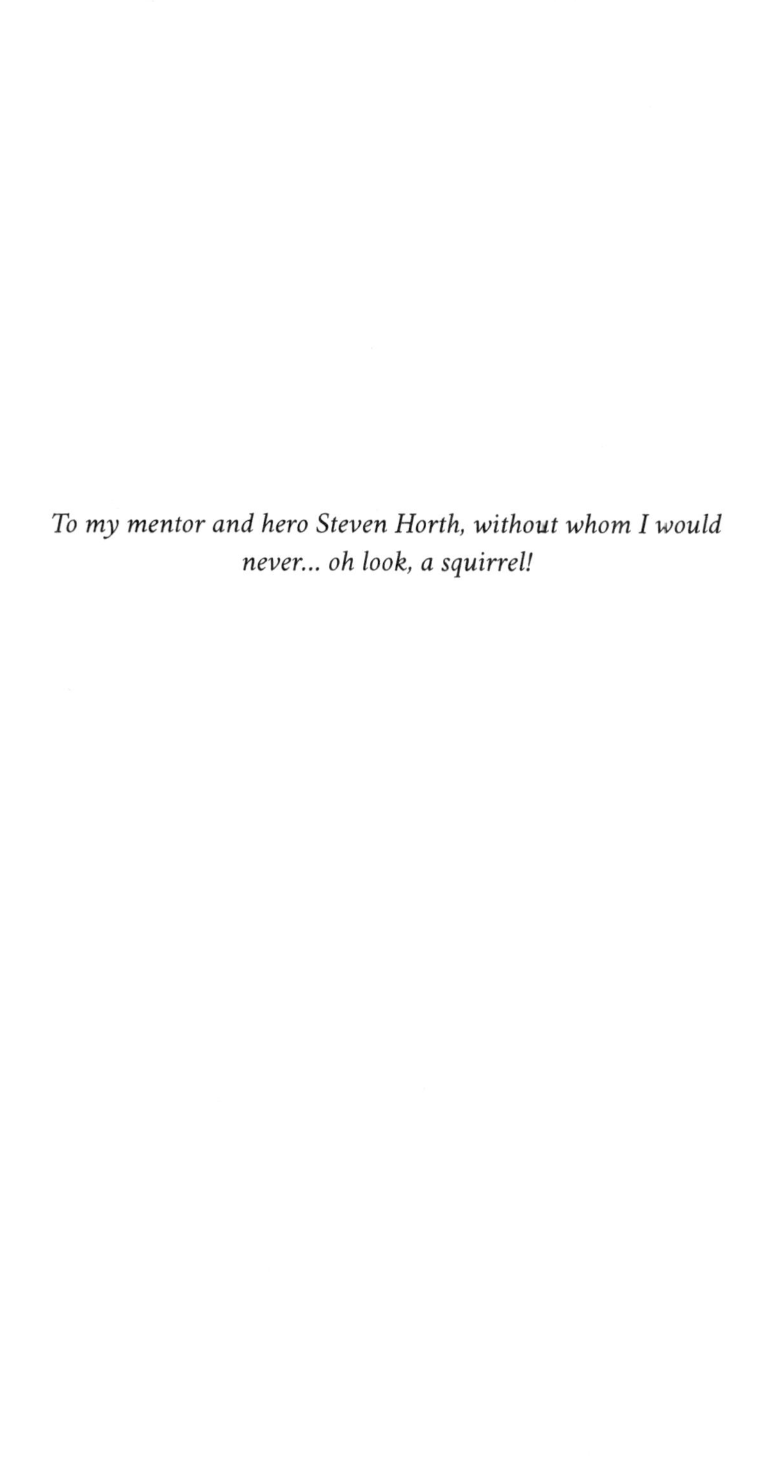

To my mentor and hero Steven Horth, without whom I would never... oh look, a squirrel!

Contents

Foreword

from Amazon.com:

Don't Give Up on Meditation!

In a world that constantly bombards us with distractions, finding inner peace and mindfulness can seem like an impossible feat. However, *"Meditation for the Easily Distracted"* offers a refreshing and accessible approach to meditation that is tailor-made for the restless mind.

Author Aubrey Dancer understands the struggles of those who find it challenging to quiet the mental chatter and maintain focus during meditation. Drawing from personal experience and years of dedicated practice, she has crafted a book that serves as a lifeline for those yearning to unlock the transformative power of meditation.

Inside the pages of *"Meditation for the Easily Distracted,"* you will discover:

Insightful Background: More than gazing into space and chanting, Dancer shows many of the various styles of mediation, as well as historical information and the various ways the Mind-Body Connection is made.

Practical Techniques: The book provides a wide range of meditation techniques, each designed to accommodate different levels of distraction. From simple breath awareness exercises to guided visualizations, you'll find methods that suit your unique needs.

Mindful Insights: Dancer shares profound insights into the nature of distraction and offers wisdom on how to navigate the turbulent waters of a restless mind. You'll learn to embrace distractions as opportunities for growth and self-awareness.

Progressive Practices: The book offers a structured path to building your meditation skills gradually. You'll start with foundational practices and gradually work your way towards deeper states of mindfulness and concentration.

Practical Tips: In addition to meditation techniques, you'll find practical tips for incorporating mindfulness into your daily life. These insights will help you stay grounded and present, even amidst life's chaos.

"Meditation for the Easily Distracted" is not just another meditation guide; it's a comprehensive and compassionate companion for anyone who has ever felt defeated by their wandering thoughts. With its gentle guidance, it empowers you to embrace your distractions and transform them into stepping stones

toward a more peaceful and centered life.

Whether you're a beginner seeking a starting point or an experienced meditator looking for fresh insights, this book will help you harness the power of meditation to navigate the modern world with calm, clarity, purpose, and focus. Get ready to embark on a journey of self-discovery and transformation like no other!

One

Introduction

Meditation describes the exact opposite of what the twenty-first century Westerner finds him/herself doing day in, day out; it also describes what we need the most to not merely survive but even thrive during these exceptionally troubling times.- Anonymous

L et us begin with a metaphor we can all relate to – a cell phone. Imagine your mind as a supercharged phone with countless apps running simultaneously. These apps represent the various things you're constantly juggling in your daily life. Here's a breakdown of some of these apps (in no particular order):

Social Media: Instagram, TikTok, Snapchat, and more. These apps are like never-ending scrolls of entertainment and social interaction. They can easily consume a lot of your attention.

Texting: You're in multiple ongoing conversations, and messages keep popping up. Each text demands a little piece of your focus.

Notifications: Your phone is constantly buzzing with notifications from various apps, alerting you to new likes, comments, messages, news updates, and more.

Multitasking: You might be doing homework, watching a YouTube video, and listening to music all at the same time. Your brain tries to manage these tasks, but it can lead to divided attention.

School and Homework: You're expected to learn and complete assignments both in school and at home. It's like having a dedicated academic app that requires your attention.

Work: Having a job can soak up your free time like nothing else!

Gaming: Video games are a massive part of many teenagers' lives. They engage your mind and can be tough to put down.

Entertainment: TV shows, movies, and streaming platforms are always available, ready to provide hours of distraction.

News and Information: You have access to an overwhelming amount of information, from news updates to educational content. It's like having an encyclopedia in your pocket.

Peer Pressure and Social Life: You want to fit in and be part of the social scene, which can add another layer of complexity to your mental landscape.

Family and Responsibilities: You have family obligations and chores, which also occupy your mental space.

Another way of thinking about these distractions would be:

Digital Devices: The proliferation of smartphones, tablets, and computers has made it easier for people to access information and entertainment at any moment. However, the constant notifications, social media updates, and a myriad of apps can easily divert attention away from important tasks.

Social Media: Social media platforms are designed to capture and hold users' attention. They offer a constant stream of new information, images, and videos, which can lead to compulsive checking and frequent interruptions throughout the day.

Multitasking: Many people believe they can efficiently juggle multiple tasks simultaneously, but in reality, true multitasking often results in reduced productivity. The brain struggles to switch between tasks, leading to errors and slower completion times.

Information Overload: The internet provides an overwhelming amount of information. People often find themselves lost in a sea of news articles, videos, and blog posts, making it difficult to focus on a single topic for an extended period.

Shortened Attention Spans: The constant exposure to quick, bite-sized content, such as tweets, memes, and short videos, has contributed to a general decrease in attention spans. It can be challenging to engage in sustained, deep thinking.

Fear of Missing Out (FOMO): The fear of missing out on something interesting or important online can drive people to keep checking their devices, even when they should be focusing on other tasks.

Stress and Anxiety: The constant barrage of information and the pressure to stay connected can lead to increased stress and anxiety levels. This, in turn, can further hinder concentration and focus.

Lack of Mindfulness: People often operate on autopilot, rushing through tasks without fully engaging with the present moment. This lack of mindfulness can contribute to a scattered mind.

Digital Addiction: Some individuals become addicted to their digital devices, spending excessive amounts of time online to the detriment of other aspects of their lives.

Environmental Distractions: Noise, interruptions, and a fast-paced lifestyle can also contribute to a distracted mind. Open office environments, for example, are notorious for creating constant interruptions and reduced concentration.

With all these concerns competing for your attention, it's easy to see why the modern distracted mind is often pulled in many directions. It can be challenging to focus on one thing for an extended period without being tempted to check your phone or switch to something more exciting. As a result, deep concentration can be hard to achieve, which can impact your productivity and ability to absorb information effectively.

It's crucial to find strategies to manage this digital distraction and allocate dedicated time for focused tasks and relaxation. We will discuss a number of strategies (*spoiler alert!*), including setting boundaries on screen time, using productivity apps to block distracting sites, or practicing mindfulness techniques to regain control of your attention. Addressing the modern distracted mind often involves intentional efforts to regain focus and mindfulness, such as practicing techniques like meditation, setting digital boundaries, and creating a conducive work environment. Additionally, recognizing the negative impacts of distraction on mental well-being and productivity is an important step toward mitigating its effects in our daily lives.

Meditation offers a wide range of physical, mental, and emotional benefits. These benefits can vary from person to person, but here are some of the most commonly reported advantages of incorporating meditation into your daily routine:

Stress Reduction: Meditation is known for its ability to reduce stress by promoting relaxation and calming the mind. It helps lower the production of stress hormones like cortisol, leading to a more balanced and peaceful state of mind. Stress which is a known risk factor for many diseases. Chronic stress can contribute to the development or exacerbation of conditions like hypertension, cardiovascular disease, and autoimmune disorders. By reducing stress, meditation may help lower the risk of these conditions.

Improved Focus and Concentration: Regular meditation practice can enhance your ability to concentrate and sustain attention. It strengthens the brain's ability to focus on tasks, which can improve productivity and performance in various aspects of life.

Emotional Well-being: Meditation can enhance emotional well-being by promoting a more positive outlook on life. It can reduce symptoms of anxiety and depression, increase feelings of happiness and contentment, and improve emotional stability. Meditation can help manage symptoms of anxiety, depression, and other mood disorders. By promoting mental well-being, meditation may indirectly contribute to better overall health outcomes.

Enhanced Cognitive Function: Some forms of meditation, such as mindfulness meditation, have been associated with improved cognitive functions like attention, memory, and problem-solving. This can be important in understanding and managing neurodegenerative diseases and cognitive disorders.

Enhanced Self-Awareness: Meditation encourages self-reflection and introspection. It helps you become more aware of your thoughts, emotions, and behaviors, leading to better understanding and self-acceptance.

Better Sleep: Many people find that meditation can improve the quality of their sleep. It can help reduce insomnia and promote more restful and rejuvenating sleep patterns. Adequate sleep is crucial for maintaining health. Meditation can help improve sleep quality and address conditions like insomnia.

Stress Management: Meditation equips you with effective stress management techniques that can be applied in daily life. It encourages a more measured response to stressful situations, reducing their impact on your overall well-being.

Pain Management: Meditation can be used as a complementary approach to managing chronic pain. By altering your perception of pain and increasing your pain tolerance, it can help alleviate discomfort to some extent. Meditation can be an effective complementary approach for managing chronic pain conditions. Understanding the potential benefits of meditation in improving pain perception and tolerance is valuable.

Improved Relationships: Enhanced emotional intelligence gained through meditation can lead to improved relationships with others. It fosters empathy, patience, and better communication skills, which can benefit both personal and professional interactions.

Boosted Immune System: Some studies suggest that meditation may have a positive impact on the immune system, potentially making you less susceptible to illnesses. Meditation can have a positive impact on the immune system. A strong immune system is essential for the body's defense against infections and diseases. Meditation may help improve immune function, making individuals more resilient to illnesses.

Inflammation Reduction: Chronic inflammation is implicated in the development of various diseases, including cancer, autoimmune disorders, and neurodegenerative conditions. Some studies suggest that meditation practices can help reduce inflammation markers in the body, potentially mitigating the risk of these diseases.

Blood Pressure Regulation: High blood pressure (hypertension) is a common risk factor for cardiovascular diseases and strokes. Meditation techniques, such as mindfulness and deep breathing, have been shown to help regulate blood pressure, which is of interest to pathologists concerned with cardiovascular health.

Spiritual Growth: For those seeking a deeper sense of spirituality or connection to a higher power, meditation can be a valuable tool. It allows for a more profound exploration of one's inner self and spirituality.

Mind-Body Connection: Meditation encourages a stronger mind-body connection, which can promote overall physical health. It can help lower blood pressure, improve cardiovascular health, and reduce the risk of various stress-related diseases.

Greater Resilience: Regular meditation practice can build mental resilience, helping you bounce back more quickly from life's challenges and setbacks.

Behavior Modification: Meditation can promote positive

lifestyle changes, such as healthier eating habits, reduced substance abuse, and increased physical activity. Pathologists can appreciate these changes as they relate to disease prevention and management.

Patient Well-Being: For medical professions working in clinical settings, understanding the benefits of meditation can lead to more comprehensive patient care. Recommending meditation as a complementary therapy may improve patients' overall well-being and recovery.

It's important to note that the benefits of meditation may take time to become noticeable, and they can vary from person to person. To experience these advantages, it's often recommended to practice meditation consistently and make it a part of your daily routine. Additionally, there are various meditation techniques, such as mindfulness meditation, loving-kindness meditation, and transcendental meditation, so you can explore different approaches to find the one that suits you best.

The bottom line is essentially this: Meditation offers a holistic approach to health and well-being, with potential benefits that can be appreciated by practitioners, our loved ones, and our healthcare professionals. By reducing stress, enhancing immune function, and improving various aspects of physical and mental health, meditation can contribute to disease prevention and the overall improvement of health outcomes.

The purpose of this book is to improve the reader's meditation experience, help easily distracted readers find focus, and cultivate mindfulness and inner calm.

Two

Understanding Distraction

Distractions (for the purposes of this discussion) are common challenges that modern people often encounter, which can hinder their ability to focus and be productive (and the effects of which can be much worse). These distractions can be broken down into two types: External distractions and Internal distractions. Here's a breakdown of these types of distractions:

External Distractions:

External distractions are factors that originate from the environment or external stimuli. They divert your attention away from your intended task. Some common external distractions in the modern world include:

Noise: Loud conversations, traffic, construction, or any other noise pollution can disrupt concentration.

Electronic Devices: Smartphones, tablets, computers, and other electronic gadgets can constantly ping with notifications, emails, and messages, tempting individuals to check them frequently.

Social Media: Social media platforms and the lure of endless scrolling through news feeds can consume a significant amount of time and attention.

Co-workers or Roommates: Interruptions from colleagues in an office setting or roommates in a shared living space can disrupt work or personal tasks.

TV and Entertainment: Television shows, video games, and streaming services provide easy access to entertainment that can pull people away from their responsibilities.

Environmental Factors: Uncomfortable room temperature, poor lighting, or an uncomfortable workspace can contribute to distraction and discomfort.

Internal Distractions:

Internal distractions stem from thoughts, feelings, or cognitive processes within an individual's mind. They can be equally, if not more, disruptive than external distractions. Common internal distractions include:

Worry and Stress: Anxiety, worries, and stress about personal issues, work-related concerns, or future events can occupy the mind and impede focus.

Daydreaming: A wandering mind that drifts away from the current task can reduce productivity.

Lack of Motivation: When individuals lack motivation or interest in a task, they are more likely to become distracted by unrelated thoughts or activities.

Multitasking: Attempting to do multiple tasks simultaneously can lead to a lack of focus on any one task, reducing overall productivity.

Procrastination: Delaying tasks or engaging in less important activities instead of completing essential tasks can be a form of self-induced distraction.

Physical Discomfort: Physical discomfort, such as hunger, tiredness, or discomfort, can be distracting and make it challenging to concentrate.

Managing external and internal distractions is essential for maintaining productivity and focus in a modern world filled with various stimuli and demands. Techniques like time management, mindfulness, setting boundaries, and creating a conducive work environment can help individuals minimize these distractions and stay on track with their tasks and goals.

How the brain processes distractions

The human brain is an incredibly complex organ responsible for processing a vast amount of information from our environment and our internal thoughts and feelings. Distractions are a common occurrence in our daily lives, and understanding how the brain processes distractions can provide valuable insights into our cognitive processes.

Perception and Sensory Input:
Distractions often start as external stimuli that enter our sensory systems. These stimuli can be visual, auditory, tactile, or even olfactory. For example, the sound of a phone ringing or a colleague's conversation nearby may grab your attention.

Selective Attention:
The brain doesn't process all incoming sensory information equally. Instead, it prioritizes certain stimuli while filtering out others. This process is called selective attention. Distractions usually occur when something unexpected or salient captures our attention and competes for cognitive resources with our current task.

Sensory Processing and Filtering:
The brain's sensory processing centers, like the primary visual or auditory cortex, initially process incoming sensory information. These regions identify the features and attributes of the stimulus. Distractions that are especially visually or auditorily stimulating may receive heightened processing at this stage.

Salience Detection:
The brain has structures like the salience network, including the anterior insula and anterior cingulate cortex, responsible for detecting the salience of stimuli. This network assesses the significance of the distraction in relation to the current task or

goal. If the distraction is deemed more salient, it's more likely to divert your attention.

Top-Down Control:

Higher-order brain regions, such as the prefrontal cortex, play a critical role in controlling attention. They maintain a cognitive framework that guides your focus. When a distraction occurs, these regions can decide whether to allocate more attention to the distraction or suppress it to maintain focus on the current task.

Working Memory and Cognitive Resources:

Working memory, located in the prefrontal cortex, is essential for holding and manipulating information temporarily. When a distraction occurs, your working memory may temporarily store information related to the distraction, pulling cognitive resources away from your primary task.

Inhibition and Suppression:

Inhibitory mechanisms in the brain help suppress distractions. The dorsolateral prefrontal cortex, for instance, is involved in inhibitory control. When you consciously decide to ignore a distraction, this region is likely involved in implementing that decision.

Reorientation of Attention:

Sometimes, a distraction might be so potent that it triggers a shift in your attention. The parietal cortex, which plays a role in spatial attention, might be involved in redirecting your focus toward the distraction.

Task Switching:

In cases where a distraction completely derails your current task, the brain may need to switch cognitive resources from your current task to address the distraction. This involves disengaging from your original task, updating your cognitive state, and engaging with the new task (the distraction).

Return to the Original Task:

After addressing the distraction or completing the secondary task, the brain must shift back to the original task. This involves reactivating the relevant cognitive processes and reestablishing focus.

The brain's ability to process distractions is a dynamic and intricate process that involves multiple regions working in concert. It's important to note that *not all distractions are processed in the same way*, as their impact on your attention can vary depending on their salience, relevance, and your cognitive state at the time. Learning to manage distractions effectively often involves *improving your ability to control attention and filter out irrelevant stimuli.*

The role of multitasking

The brain is a complex organ capable of performing numerous tasks simultaneously, although it's important to note that the term "multitasking" can be somewhat misleading when applied to the brain. Instead of true parallel processing like a computer, the brain efficiently switches its focus between different tasks and processes in a rapid and seamless manner. This dynamic ability to manage various functions simultaneously and switch between them is sometimes referred to as "task switching" or "parallel processing."

Here's a breakdown of how the brain multitasks:

Parallel Processing: The brain is divided into different regions and networks responsible for various functions such as vision, hearing, memory, motor skills, language, and emotions. These regions can operate simultaneously, allowing you to perform multiple functions at once. For example, you can walk and talk or listen to music while driving.

Task Switching: The brain is exceptionally skilled at quickly shifting its attention between tasks. This ability allows you to switch from one activity to another seamlessly. For instance, you can read a book, answer a phone call, and then return to your book without much difficulty.

Cognitive Flexibility: Multitasking involves cognitive flexibility, which allows the brain to adapt to new situations and tasks. This includes adjusting your focus, priorities, and mental resources as needed.

Automatic Processes: Many everyday activities become automatic with practice and repetition. These automatic processes require minimal cognitive effort, freeing up mental resources for other tasks. For example, skilled musicians can play complex pieces without thinking about every individual note.

Working Memory: Working memory is a temporary storage system that allows you to hold and manipulate information briefly. It plays a crucial role in multitasking by allowing you to keep track of different tasks simultaneously. For example, when you mentally calculate a tip while ordering food, you're using working memory.

Attention Control: The brain can allocate attention selectively to different stimuli or tasks. This helps you focus on the most important or urgent task at any given moment while temporarily setting aside less important ones.

Prioritization: The brain constantly assesses the importance of different tasks and allocates resources accordingly. This prioritization helps you manage your time and make decisions about which tasks to focus on.

Limitations: While the brain is incredibly adept at multitasking, it has limitations. Attempting to handle too many tasks simultaneously can lead to decreased performance, increased stress, and mental fatigue. Some tasks require intense concentration and cannot be effectively multitasked.

To put it all together, the brain's ability to multitask involves a combination of parallel processing, task switching, cognitive flexibility, automatic processes, working memory, attention control, and prioritization. While it can handle multiple tasks at once, it is essential to recognize its limitations and the potential negative effects of overloading it with too many simultaneous tasks. Effective time management and task prioritization are key to optimizing the brain's multitasking capabilities.

The Cost of Chronic Distraction

Chronic (non-temporary) distraction can have a significant impact on both productivity and mental health. In today's digital age, where we are constantly bombarded with information and notifications, it's increasingly common for people to struggle with chronic distraction. Here are some of the ways it can affect productivity and mental health:

Reduced Productivity:

a. Decreased Focus: Chronic distractions can make it difficult to concentrate on tasks, leading to reduced focus and attention. This can result in errors, missed deadlines, and lower-quality work.

b. Task Switching: Constantly shifting attention between tasks or responding to interruptions can disrupt workflow and lead to inefficiency. It takes time to regain focus after each distraction, further decreasing productivity.

c. Procrastination: Distractions can provide an easy escape from challenging or tedious tasks, encouraging procrastination. This can lead to a backlog of work and increased stress.

Increased Stress and Anxiety:

a. Information Overload: The constant stream of information from emails, social media, and other sources can lead to information overload. This can create feelings of overwhelm and stress.

b. Multitasking Stress: Juggling multiple tasks due to distractions can result in increased stress and anxiety as you try to keep up with various demands simultaneously.

c. Fear of Missing Out (FOMO): Frequent distractions can lead to a fear of missing out on important information or opportunities, causing anxiety and compulsive checking of notifications.

d. Reduced Work-Life Balance: Chronic distraction can spill over into personal time, leading to a blurred boundary between work and leisure, which can contribute to burnout.

Impaired Cognitive Function:

a. Reduced Memory: Distractions can interfere with the encoding and retrieval of information, making it harder to remember important details and tasks.

b. Impaired Decision-Making: A distracted mind is less likely to make well-informed decisions, potentially leading to poor choices in both personal and professional life.

Decreased Job Satisfaction:

a. Lack of Accomplishment: Chronic distraction can prevent individuals from feeling a sense of accomplishment at work, which is crucial for job satisfaction and motivation.

b. Decreased Engagement: Constant distractions can hinder engagement with tasks, making work feel less meaningful and enjoyable.

Negative Impact on Relationships:

a. Reduced Presence: Chronic distraction can affect personal relationships, as individuals may be physically present but mentally absent when spending time with loved ones.

b. Communication Breakdown: Frequent interruptions and divided attention can lead to communication problems and misunderstandings in both personal and professional relationships.

To mitigate the impact of chronic distraction on productivity and mental health, individuals can adopt strategies such as time management techniques, setting boundaries with digital devices, creating distraction-free work environments, and practicing mindfulness. Employers can also support their employees by promoting a healthy work-life balance, providing training on distraction management, and fostering a culture of focus and productivity. Ultimately, addressing chronic distraction requires a combination of personal awareness and systemic changes to create a more conducive environment for sustained attention and well-being.

Three

The Basics of Meditation

Definitions and Misconceptions

Sometimes our misconceptions about meditation itself are enough to distract us to failure! So, let's define our terms:

Meditation is a mental practice: Meditation is a mental exercise that involves focusing your attention on a particular object, thought, or activity to train the mind and achieve a state of mental clarity, relaxation, or heightened awareness.

Mindfulness Meditation: This form of meditation involves paying non-judgmental attention to the present moment. It often involves observing your thoughts, feelings, and bodily sensations as they arise without trying to change or judge them.

Concentration Meditation: In this type of meditation, you focus your attention on a single point, such as your breath, a mantra, or a candle flame. The goal is to cultivate deep concentration and mental stability.

Loving-Kindness Meditation (Metta): This practice involves generating feelings of compassion, love, and goodwill towards oneself and others. It aims to cultivate a sense of interconnectedness and promote positive emotions.

Transcendental Meditation: A specific technique where you repeat a specific mantra silently. It is designed to lead to a state of restful awareness and deep relaxation.

Common Misconceptions about Meditation:

Meditation is about emptying your mind: This is a prevalent misconception. While some forms of meditation may involve quieting the mind, the goal is not to completely empty it. Instead, it's about directing and sustaining your focus on a chosen point of attention.

Meditation is religious: Meditation can be practiced within a religious context, but it's not inherently tied to any religion. Many people use meditation as a secular practice for stress reduction, self-improvement, or mental well-being.

Meditation requires sitting in a lotus position: While the lotus position is a traditional meditation posture, it's not necessary for everyone. Meditation can be done while sitting in a chair, lying down, or even walking. The key is to find a comfortable and stable posture that works for you.

Meditation is an escape from reality: Meditation is not about escaping from reality but rather about developing a deeper awareness of reality as it is. It can help you better understand and respond to the challenges and stressors in your life.

Meditation brings instant enlightenment or relaxation: While some people may experience immediate benefits from meditation, it often takes time and consistent practice to see significant results. Patience and regularity are key to reaping the long-term benefits.

You have to stop thinking during meditation: It's normal for thoughts to arise during meditation. The goal is not to eliminate thoughts but to observe them without attachment and gently redirect your focus to your chosen point of attention.

Meditation is only for people with a calm mind: Meditation can be especially beneficial for people with busy or anxious minds. It can help calm and clarify the mind over time, but it's not reserved for those who already have a calm disposition.

Meditation is only for experienced practitioners: Anyone can start meditating, regardless of their experience level. There are many beginner-friendly meditation techniques and resources available to help you get started.

Basically, meditation is a diverse practice with various forms and purposes, and it doesn't necessarily conform to many of the common misconceptions. It's essential to approach meditation with an open mind and a willingness to learn and adapt to your own needs and preferences.

————————————-

Meditation has a rich and diverse historical context that spans thousands of years and is deeply rooted in various cultures and traditions around the world. While it's challenging to provide an exhaustive overview of meditation's entire history, I can offer a general overview of its historical development and key milestones in different regions and cultures.

Prehistoric and Indigenous Practices:
Meditation likely has its origins in prehistoric times, with evidence of meditative practices found in ancient cave paintings and artifacts. Indigenous cultures across the globe have also practiced forms of meditation as a means of connecting with nature, ancestors, and the spiritual world.

Ancient India:
One of the earliest documented accounts of meditation comes from ancient India, where it played a central role in the development of Hinduism. The ancient texts known as the Vedas (c. 1500-500 BCE) mention meditation practices aimed at achieving spiritual insight and liberation (moksha).

Buddhism:
Siddhartha Gautama, later known as the Buddha, is a pivotal figure in the history of meditation. Around the 5th century BCE, he developed a systematic approach to meditation as a means to attain enlightenment (nirvana). The Four Noble

Truths and the Eightfold Path included meditation as a fundamental practice in Buddhism.

Taoism:

In ancient China, Taoism emphasized meditation as a way to align with the natural order (Tao). Taoist meditation practices often involved breath control, visualization, and movement, as seen in Tai Chi and Qigong.

Ancient Greece:

The Hellenistic period saw the rise of philosophical schools like Stoicism and Epicureanism that incorporated meditative practices into their teachings. The philosopher Plotinus developed a form of meditation called "Enneads," which influenced later Western mystical traditions.

Islamic Sufism:

Sufism, a mystical branch of Islam, has a long history of incorporating meditation and contemplative practices. Sufi mystics sought to deepen their connection with Allah through techniques like dhikr (repetitive chanting) and inward reflection.

Old and New Testament:

Meditation has a long history in Judaism and Christianity. While the practice of meditation as it's commonly understood today may not be explicitly mentioned in the Bible, there are several biblical references and passages that allude to contemplative and meditative practices. Here are some notable references:

Psalm 1:2: *"But his delight is in the law of the Lord, and on his law, he meditates day and night."* This verse suggests the importance of meditating on God's word as a source of joy and spiritual growth.

Psalm 19:14: *"May the words of my mouth and the meditation of my heart be pleasing to you, O Lord, my rock and my redeemer."* Here, the psalmist expresses the desire for their thoughts and inner reflections to be in alignment with God's will.

Psalm 119:15: *"I will meditate on your [God's] precepts and fix my eyes on your ways."* This verse emphasizes the act of meditating on God's commandments as a way to better understand and follow them.

Joshua 1:8: *"This Book of the Law shall not depart from your mouth, but you shall meditate on it day and night, so that you may be careful to do according to all that is written in it. For then you will make your way prosperous, and then you will have good success."* Joshua is instructed to meditate on the Book of the Law as a means to ensure success and obedience.

Philippians 4:8: *"Finally, brothers, whatever is true, whatever is honorable, whatever is just, whatever is pure, whatever is lovely, whatever is commendable, if there is any excellence, if there is anything worthy of praise, think about these things."* While not explicitly meditation, this verse encourages believers to focus their thoughts on virtuous and positive things, which aligns with the essence of meditation.

1 Timothy 4:15: *"Practice these things, immerse yourself in them*

so that all may see your progress." This verse suggests immersing oneself deeply in spiritual practices, which typically includes meditation and contemplation.

It's important to note that the concept of meditation in the Bible may differ from Eastern meditation practices in some aspects. Biblical meditation often involves focused reflection on God's word, prayer, and seeking a deeper connection with God. It is a way to align one's thoughts and heart with divine wisdom and guidance.

Christian Mysticism:
Christian mystics, such as the Desert Fathers and Mothers in the early Christian era, practiced meditation and contemplation to deepen their relationship with God. This tradition later evolved into Christian contemplative practices and monastic traditions.

Medieval Japan:
Zen Buddhism, which originated in China but became particularly influential in Japan during the medieval period, emphasized meditation (zazen) as the primary means of attaining enlightenment. Zen's simplicity and direct approach to meditation had a significant impact on Japanese culture.

Modern Era:
In the 20th century, meditation gained popularity in the West through figures like Paramahansa Yogananda, who introduced Yoga and meditation to Western audiences. The 1960s saw a surge in interest in meditation due to cultural exchange with Eastern spirituality and the work of figures like Maharishi

Mahesh Yogi and the Beatles.

Contemporary Meditation:
Today, meditation has become a global phenomenon, with various traditions and secular forms of meditation widely practiced. Mindfulness meditation, Vipassana, Transcendental Meditation, and many others have gained popularity for their potential benefits to mental and emotional well-being.

Meditation's historical context is multifaceted, reflecting the diverse spiritual and philosophical traditions from which it emerged. Over time, it has evolved and adapted, taking on different forms and purposes across cultures and generations. In the modern era, meditation continues to evolve as scientific research explores its potential benefits for physical and mental health.

The Mind-Body Connection:
The mind-body connection is a complex and multifaceted concept in psychology that refers to the interrelationship between a person's mental and emotional state (the "mind") and their physical health and well-being (the "body"). Psychologists study this connection to better understand how our thoughts, emotions, and behaviors can influence our physical health and vice versa. There are several key aspects to consider when exploring the mind-body connection from a psychological perspective:

Psychosomatic Effects: Psychologists have long recognized that psychological factors can have a significant impact on physical health. For example, stress, anxiety, and depression can contribute to the development or exacerbation of physical illnesses. These connections are often referred to as "psychosomatic" effects.

Stress Response: The body's stress response is a prime example of the mind-body connection. When a person perceives a threat or experiences stress, the brain initiates a series of physiological responses, such as increased heart rate, elevated blood pressure, and the release of stress hormones like cortisol. Over time, chronic stress can contribute to a range of health problems, including cardiovascular disease, digestive disorders, and weakened immune function.

Placebo and Nocebo Effects: Psychologists also study how a person's beliefs and expectations can influence their physical health. The placebo effect occurs when a person experiences improvements in their symptoms or condition after receiving a treatment that has no active therapeutic ingredient simply because they believe it will work. Conversely, the nocebo effect can lead to negative outcomes when a person expects harm or side effects from a treatment.

Mind-Body Interventions: Psychologists and healthcare providers often employ mind-body interventions as part of holistic approaches to health and wellness. These interventions include practices like mindfulness meditation, yoga, biofeedback, and relaxation techniques. These practices aim to promote mental and emotional well-being while also improving physical health by reducing stress, enhancing immune function, and improving pain management.

Health Behavior Change: Psychologists play a crucial role in helping individuals make positive health behavior changes. This includes addressing issues like smoking cessation, diet, exercise, and medication adherence. Understanding the psychology of motivation, self-control, and habit formation is essential in promoting healthier behaviors and improved physical health.

Emotions and Physical Health: Psychologists investigate how emotions can impact physical health. For instance, chronic anger or hostility has been linked to an increased risk of heart disease. Positive emotions, on the other hand, can contribute to better physical health outcomes, such as enhanced immune function and quicker recovery from illness.

Mind-Body Medicine: In the field of mind-body medicine, psychologists collaborate with healthcare providers to integrate psychological interventions into medical treatment plans. This may involve helping patients manage pain, cope with chronic illnesses, or improve their overall well-being through psychological techniques.

————————————-

Stepping away from the purely physical/emotional realm, a spiritualist would have a fundamentally different (and valuable) view that we can examine here:

From the perspective of a spiritualist, the mind-body connection is deeply intertwined and goes beyond the purely physical and materialistic explanations offered by conventional science. Spiritualists believe that the mind and body are interconnected in a holistic and metaphysical way, and this connection is crucial for understanding human existence and well-being. Here are some key concepts related to the mind-body connection from a spiritualist point of view:

Energy and Vibrations: Spiritualists often emphasize the concept of energy and vibrations as the underlying forces that connect the mind and body. They believe that everything, including our thoughts and emotions, emits energy and vibrations that influence our physical and mental state.

Chakras and Energy Centers: Spiritualists frequently refer to the existence of energy centers within the body, known as chakras. These chakras are believed to be hubs of spiritual and emotional energy, and their balance or imbalance can affect both physical health and mental well-being.

Thoughts Create Reality: Spiritualists often subscribe to the idea that our thoughts have the power to shape our reality. They believe that positive thoughts and intentions can lead to positive outcomes in both the physical and spiritual realms, while negative thoughts can have detrimental effects.

Emotions and Physical Health: Spiritualists recognize the strong connection between emotions and physical health. They believe that repressed emotions or unresolved emotional issues can manifest as physical illnesses or ailments.

Meditation and Mindfulness: Practices such as meditation and mindfulness are frequently recommended by spiritualists to strengthen the mind-body connection. These practices are seen as a means of aligning one's thoughts and emotions with their physical well-being and spiritual growth.

Holistic Healing: Spiritualists often seek holistic approaches to healing that consider the whole person, including their physical, mental, emotional, and spiritual aspects. This may involve alternative therapies like energy healing, acupuncture, or herbal medicine.

Reincarnation and Karma: Some spiritual traditions believe in the concept of reincarnation and karma, where the experiences and actions of the mind and body in one lifetime can have repercussions in future lifetimes. This perspective underscores the idea that the mind and body are interconnected across different lifetimes.

Intuition and Psychic Abilities: Spiritualists often believe in the existence of intuitive and psychic abilities, which they see as a manifestation of the mind's connection to a higher spiritual realm. These abilities are believed to provide insights into the interconnectedness of all things.

Spiritual Growth and Enlightenment: Ultimately, spiritualists view the mind-body connection as a path to spiritual growth and enlightenment. They believe that by nurturing this connection and aligning with higher spiritual truths, individuals can achieve a deeper understanding of themselves and their place in the universe.

It's important to note that the perspectives of spiritualists can vary widely depending on their specific beliefs and practices. While these concepts provide an overview of how a spiritualist might view the mind-body connection, individual interpretations and beliefs within the spiritualist community can differ significantly.

In summary, the mind-body connection is a critical area of study within psychology that examines the bidirectional relationship between mental and emotional well-being and physical health. Understanding this connection can lead to improved health outcomes and a more holistic approach to healthcare. Psychologists use a variety of methods and interventions to explore and address the mind-body connection, ultimately aiming to enhance both mental and physical well-being.

———————————-

A holistic approach to meditation involves considering the interconnectedness of the mind, body, and spirit, and it emphasizes the integration of various meditation techniques and practices to promote overall well-being. This approach recognizes that our mental, emotional, and physical states are interconnected, and by addressing them simultaneously, we can achieve a more profound and lasting sense of balance and harmony. Here are some benefits of adopting a holistic approach to meditation:

Improved Physical Health:
Stress Reduction: Holistic meditation techniques can help reduce stress, which is linked to various health problems like

hypertension, cardiovascular disease, and weakened immune function.

Pain Management: Meditation can be effective in managing chronic pain conditions by promoting relaxation and reducing the perception of pain.

Better Sleep: Holistic meditation practices can improve sleep quality and help with insomnia by calming the mind and reducing anxiety.

Enhanced Emotional Well-Being:

Emotional Regulation: Holistic meditation fosters emotional awareness and helps individuals better understand and regulate their emotions, leading to improved emotional resilience.

Reduced Anxiety and Depression: Meditation can be a valuable tool in reducing symptoms of anxiety and depression by promoting relaxation and enhancing mood.

Mental Clarity and Focus:

Increased Concentration: Holistic meditation practices often include mindfulness techniques that improve concentration and cognitive function, which can benefit work and daily tasks.

Enhanced Creativity: A holistic approach to meditation can stimulate creativity by quieting the mind and allowing for the free flow of ideas.

Spiritual Growth and Connection:

Deepened Sense of Purpose: For those seeking a spiritual dimension, holistic meditation can provide a deeper sense of purpose and connection to something greater than themselves.

Self-Discovery: Holistic meditation practices often encourage self-reflection and self-discovery, allowing individuals to explore their beliefs, values, and inner wisdom.

Better Relationships:

Improved Communication: Meditation can enhance communication skills by increasing empathy, active listening, and emotional intelligence, which can lead to healthier relationships.

Reduced Conflict: Holistic meditation can help individuals respond more skillfully to conflicts and challenges, reducing interpersonal conflicts.

Holistic Healing:

Mind-Body Connection: Holistic meditation acknowledges the mind-body connection and how our mental state can influence physical health, allowing for a more comprehensive approach to healing.

Integrative Approach: Holistic meditation can complement conventional medical treatments, promoting overall healing and well-being.

Stress Resilience:

Coping Skills: By practicing meditation regularly, individuals can develop better coping skills, enabling them to navigate life's challenges with greater resilience.

Long-term Well-Being:

Sustainable Change: Holistic meditation encourages a long-term commitment to well-being, as it addresses various aspects of health and personal growth simultaneously.

In summary, a holistic approach to meditation offers a wide range of benefits by recognizing the interconnectedness of our mental, emotional, and physical states. It promotes overall well-being, helping individuals achieve balance and harmony in their lives. Whether you are seeking stress reduction, emotional balance, improved physical health, or spiritual growth, a holistic approach to meditation can be a valuable tool in your journey towards well-being and self-discovery.

————————————————-

Designing a distraction-free meditation space

Creating a distraction-free environment for meditation is essential to help you achieve a deep and focused practice. A serene and undisturbed space can enhance your mindfulness and make it easier to cultivate inner peace. Here are some key considerations and tips for designing a distraction-free environment for meditation:

Choose a Quiet Location:

Find a quiet room or corner of your home where you are less likely to be disturbed by external noises like traffic, conversations, or electronic devices.

Consider using earplugs or white noise machines if external sounds are unavoidable.

Declutter the Space:

Remove unnecessary items from your meditation area. A clutter-free environment can help create a sense of calm and reduce visual distractions.

Keep the space clean and organized to promote a peaceful

atmosphere.

Comfortable Seating:

Select a comfortable and supportive cushion or chair for meditation. The goal is to maintain good posture without discomfort.

Ensure the seating arrangement promotes proper alignment of your back and neck to avoid physical distractions during your practice.

Proper Lighting:

Soft, diffused, and natural lighting is ideal for meditation. Consider using curtains or blinds to control the amount of light in the room.

Candlelight or low-level ambient lighting can create a soothing atmosphere.

Temperature Control:

Maintain a comfortable temperature in the room. Being too hot or too cold can be distracting during meditation.

Use blankets or shawls to regulate your body temperature as needed.

Aromatherapy:

Some people find that using essential oils or incense can enhance their meditation experience by creating a pleasant aroma in the space.

Choose scents that promote relaxation, such as lavender, sandalwood, or frankincense.

Minimal Decor:

Keep the decoration minimal and purposeful. A few calming images or symbols, such as a Buddha statue or a serene painting, can be inspiring without being distracting.

Avoid visually stimulating or busy artwork.

Turn Off Electronics:

Power down or silence all electronic devices like phones, tablets, and computers to eliminate potential distractions from notifications and sounds.

Consider using a dedicated meditation timer or app on airplane mode if you require a timer.

Create Rituals:

Establish a meditation routine with a simple ritual that helps signal the beginning and end of your practice. This can be lighting a candle, ringing a bell, or taking a few deep breaths.

Consistency in your meditation rituals can train your mind to enter a focused state more easily.

Inform Others:

Let family members or roommates know your meditation schedule so they can respect your quiet time and avoid disturbing you.

Personalize Your Space:

Customize your meditation environment to suit your preferences. What matters most is that it feels peaceful and conducive to your practice.

Remember that creating a distraction-free environment is just one aspect of successful meditation. Ultimately, the most important factors are your commitment, regular practice, and the development of mindfulness techniques that allow you to remain focused even in less-than-ideal conditions.

Over time, you may find that you become less affected by external distractions, both during meditation and in your daily life.

Meditation and mindfulness

Meditation and mindfulness are related practices that often overlap but have distinct differences in their focus, techniques, and goals. Here are the key differences between meditation and mindfulness:

Definition:

Meditation: Meditation is a broad term that encompasses various techniques and practices designed to cultivate a state of focused attention, relaxation, and heightened awareness. It often involves directing your thoughts and concentration in a specific way, which can include mantra repetition, breath awareness, or visualization.

Mindfulness: Mindfulness is a specific type of meditation but can also be thought of as a broader way of approaching daily life. Mindfulness involves paying non-judgmental attention to the present moment, observing your thoughts, feelings, sensations, and surroundings without trying to change or judge them.

Technique:

Meditation: In meditation, the focus is often on a single point of attention, such as your breath, a mantra, or a visual object. The goal is to quiet the mind, reduce mental chatter, and achieve a deep state of concentration or relaxation.

Mindfulness: Mindfulness involves maintaining an open awareness of whatever is happening in the present moment. This can be done during everyday activities, such as eating, walking, or simply sitting quietly. Rather than narrowing your focus, mindfulness broadens it to include everything you're experiencing without attachment or aversion.

Purpose:

Meditation: The goals of meditation can vary widely depending on the specific practice. Some common purposes include stress reduction, improving concentration, gaining insight into the self, or achieving spiritual growth. Meditation can be goal-oriented.

Mindfulness: The primary purpose of mindfulness is to cultivate awareness and acceptance of the present moment, without any specific agenda or outcome. It is often used as a tool for managing stress, enhancing well-being and increasing emotional intelligence.

Time Commitment:

Meditation: Meditation sessions can vary in length, ranging from a few minutes to hours, depending on the specific technique and the individual's preference. Some people engage in daily meditation practices, while others do it less frequently.

Mindfulness: Mindfulness can be practiced throughout the day, even in short moments of focused awareness during daily activities. Formal mindfulness meditation sessions are typically shorter and can be integrated into one's daily routine more easily.

Application:
Meditation: Meditation practices are often used as a specific activity, typically done while sitting or lying down, with the aim of achieving a particular state of consciousness.

Mindfulness: Mindfulness can be applied to various aspects of life, from eating and walking to working and interacting with others. It's about being fully present and engaged in whatever you are doing.

Spiritual vs. Secular:
Meditation: Many meditation practices have spiritual or religious roots and are used for spiritual development and enlightenment. However, secular meditation practices also exist, which focus on mental well-being and stress reduction.

Mindfulness: While mindfulness has its roots in Buddhist meditation, it has been widely secularized and adapted for therapeutic and stress-reduction purposes in non-religious contexts.

In summary, meditation and mindfulness are related practices, but meditation is a broader category that includes various techniques and goals, while mindfulness is a specific form of meditation focused on cultivating present-moment awareness and acceptance. Both can be valuable tools for enhancing mental and emotional well-being, and individuals may choose the one that aligns best with their goals and preferences.

— — — — — — — — — —

Incorporating mindfulness into daily life

Incorporating mindfulness into daily life involves *cultivating a state of active awareness and presence in each moment.* Mindfulness is a practice rooted in ancient Buddhist traditions but has gained significant popularity in recent years due to its numerous mental, emotional, and physical health benefits. Here are some practical ways to integrate mindfulness into your daily routine:

Start with the Breath: The breath is a powerful anchor for mindfulness. Begin your day by taking a few moments to focus on your breath. Simply observe the inhales and exhales without judgment. This can set a positive tone for the day.

Morning Routine: Transform your morning routine into a mindfulness practice. Pay attention to the sensations of brushing your teeth, showering, or having breakfast. Engage fully in these activities rather than letting your mind wander.

Mindful Eating: Instead of rushing through meals or eating while distracted, savor each bite. Pay attention to the flavors, textures, and smells of your food. Eating mindfully can also help with portion control and overeating.

Walking Meditation: Incorporate mindfulness into your daily walk, whether it's a leisurely stroll or a commute. Focus on the sensation of each step and your connection with the ground. Notice the sights and sounds around you.

Mindful Technology Use: Be conscious of how you use

technology. Limit multitasking, and when using your devices, do so with intention. Turn off notifications and take breaks to check in with yourself.

Mindful Breathing Breaks: Throughout the day, take short breaks to focus on your breath. A few minutes of deep, mindful breathing can reduce stress and improve concentration.

Mindful Listening: When talking to someone, practice active listening. Give them your full attention without thinking about what you'll say next. This can improve relationships and communication.

Mindful Work: Apply mindfulness at work by giving your full attention to the task at hand. Avoid multitasking, and take short breaks to clear your mind and refocus.

Mindful Body Scan: Take a few minutes to scan your body for tension or discomfort. This can help you become aware of physical sensations and reduce stress.

Evening Reflection: Before bed, reflect on your day. Acknowledge your thoughts, emotions, and experiences without judgment. This can help you let go of stress and prepare for a restful night's sleep.

Mindful Gratitude: Cultivate gratitude by taking a moment each day to acknowledge the things you're thankful for. This can foster a positive mindset and increase overall well-being.

Mindful Communication: When engaging in conversations,

be aware of your words and their impact. Practice compassionate and empathetic communication.

Mindfulness Apps and Resources: There are numerous mindfulness apps and guided meditations available that can help you develop and maintain a regular mindfulness practice.

Remember that mindfulness is a skill that takes time to develop. Be patient with yourself and approach it with a non-judgmental attitude. Over time, incorporating mindfulness into your daily life can lead to increased self-awareness, reduced stress, enhanced emotional regulation, and an overall sense of well-being.

Four

Meditation Techniques for the Easily Distracted

For many of you, you've probably fast-forwarded passed the previous chapters, hoping to get to the meat of this content – *how do I eliminate the distractions I experience when I (try to) meditate?*

I don't blame you! If that is you, I urge you to go back and read through the beginning parts of this book *when you have some free time.* It probably isn't critical information for what you specifically are going through, but it would be helpful down the line.

I've included quite a bit of scientific and medical information in this book for a few reasons.

First, I'm a **total geek** when it comes to that stuff.

Second, much of the distraction I personally experienced had to do with my total ignorance of all things Meditation. You, gentle reader, should not have that excuse now!

The Distraction Sink (*this will take some work*):

To over-simplify things, there are two ways of dealing with distractions as they happen: One way is to immediately decide this is *trivial/stupid/evil and I need pay no more attention to it.* Fine. Blocking that is what the rest of this book is about.

The other way is to decide *this is important but I need to deal with it later.* I recommend having a notepad handy where the process of writing it down and knowing *you will absolutely address this later today* releases it from your immediate concern and lets you move on to meditation.

If you are concerned that an issue needs to be addressed and it will probably leap into your brain when you don't want it to, I would strongly suggest you either postpone meditation and deal with it first or add an hour to your proverbial calendar when you will deal with it.

And again, you have to absolutely without fail know in your deepest innermost being that you effing *will deal with it then.* If you have doubts, those doubts will want to interfere with your meditation.

You need to develop a reputation with yourself (I'll give you a minute to wrap your brain around that) that you are perfectly dependable when you give your Sacred Word that this issue that isn't easily going away will in fact be handled shortly and you absolutely know this because you've given your Sacred Word in the past about similar issues and you have ALWAYS kept your Word! (wink wink)

Now you've taken that distraction and locked it away for the time being, making it no longer part of the picture.

I know, much easier said than done.

Now, on with the show:

Mindfulness Meditation

Breathing exercises are a fundamental aspect of meditation, as they help calm the mind, increase mindfulness, and enhance relaxation. Here are some useful breathing exercises for meditation:

Deep Abdominal Breathing (Diaphragmatic Breathing):
Sit or lie down in a comfortable position.
Place one hand on your chest and the other on your abdomen.
Inhale deeply through your nose, allowing your abdomen to rise as you fill your lungs.
Exhale slowly and completely through your mouth, feeling your abdomen fall.
Focus your attention on the rise and fall of your abdomen and the rhythm of your breath.

Counted Breath:
In a comfortable meditation posture, inhale slowly and deeply through your nose to a count of four.
Hold your breath for a count of four.
Exhale slowly and completely through your mouth to a count of six.

Repeat this cycle, gradually increasing the count as you become more comfortable.

4-7-8 Breathing (Relaxing Breath):

Sit in a relaxed position with your back straight.

Close your eyes and inhale quietly through your nose for a count of four.

Hold your breath for a count of seven.

Exhale completely and audibly through your mouth for a count of eight.

Repeat this cycle for several rounds.

Alternate Nostril Breathing (Nadi Shodhana):

Sit in a comfortable position with your spine straight.

Use your right thumb to close off your right nostril and your right ring finger to close off your left nostril.

Close your eyes and inhale deeply through your left nostril.

Close off your left nostril with your ring finger, release your right nostril, and exhale through your right nostril.

Inhale through your right nostril, close it off, release your left nostril, and exhale through your left nostril.

This completes one round. Repeat for several rounds.

Box Breathing (Square Breathing):

Sit comfortably and close your eyes.

Inhale through your nose for a count of four.

Hold your breath for a count of four.

Exhale through your mouth for a count of four.

Hold your breath for another count of four.

Repeat this pattern for several rounds, creating a square shape with your breath.

Body Scan Breathing:

Start at the top of your head and progressively focus on each body part as you breathe.

As you inhale, visualize warm, soothing energy entering that body part.

As you exhale, imagine tension and stress leaving that body part.

Move downward through your body, scanning and relaxing each part.

Mantra Breathing:

Choose a calming word or phrase (a mantra) and silently repeat it with each breath.

Inhale while silently saying the first part of the mantra, and exhale while saying the second part.

This helps keep your mind focused and calm during meditation.

Remember that the key to successful meditation is consistency and patience. Start with shorter sessions and gradually increase the duration as you become more comfortable with these breathing exercises. The goal is to cultivate a sense of inner peace, presence, and mindfulness through your breath.

Resources:

Using audio and visual aids can be helpful when meditating, as they can enhance your meditation experience and deepen your practice. These aids can help you focus, relax, and reach a state of mindfulness more effectively. Here are some ways you can use audio and visual aids in meditation:

Guided Meditation:

Audio: Guided meditation recordings or apps can provide you with a voice to lead you through a meditation session. A trained meditation instructor or soothing voice can help you stay on track and provide guidance on various meditation techniques.

Visual: You can follow along with guided meditation videos that offer both audio and visual cues. These videos may include calming visuals, such as nature scenes or soothing animations, to enhance your meditation experience.

Binaural Beats and Brainwave Entrainment:

Audio: Binaural beats are auditory illusions created when you listen to two slightly different frequencies in each ear. They can help induce specific brainwave states, such as relaxation or deep focus, which can complement your meditation practice.

Visual: Some apps or videos combine binaural beats with visual elements like pulsating light patterns. These can be used to synchronize your brainwaves and deepen your meditative experience.

Music and Soundscapes:

Audio: Soft, instrumental music or ambient sounds, like flowing water, bird chirping, or gentle rain, can create a serene atmosphere for meditation. Choose music or sounds that resonate with you and promote relaxation.

Visual: You can pair calming visuals with music or sound-scapes to enhance the overall sensory experience. These visuals could include scenes of nature or abstract patterns that promote tranquility.

Mantras and Affirmations:

Audio: Repeating a mantra or affirmation, either silently or out loud, can help focus your mind during meditation. You can find audio recordings of mantras or affirmations to assist you in your practice.

Visual: You can display written mantras or affirmations in your meditation space or use visualization techniques to enhance their impact during your practice.

Mindfulness Apps and Virtual Reality:

Audio: Many mindfulness apps offer a variety of meditation sessions with audio guidance, timers, and progress tracking. These apps can be especially useful for beginners.

Visual: Virtual reality (VR) meditation experiences can immerse you in a visually stimulating environment, making it easier to detach from distractions and immerse yourself in your meditation practice.

Candle Gazing and Mandalas:

Visual: Candle gazing involves focusing on the flame of a candle, while mandalas are intricate geometric patterns to meditate upon. These visual aids can help improve concentration and inner peace during meditation.

When using audio and visual aids in meditation, it's essential to choose what resonates with you personally and aligns with your meditation goals. Experiment with different aids to find the ones that enhance your practice and contribute to your overall sense of well-being and mindfulness. Remember that the ultimate goal of meditation is to cultivate inner awareness and stillness, and these aids are tools to assist you in achieving that state.

Movement-Based Meditation

Movement-based meditation, also known as mindfulness in motion or embodied meditation, is a form of meditation that combines physical movement with mindfulness techniques. While traditional seated meditation involves stillness and focusing on the breath or a specific point of concentration, movement-based meditation encourages mindfulness and presence while in motion. Here are some advantages of practicing movement-based meditation:

Physical Health Benefits:

Improved Flexibility: Many movement-based meditation practices involve gentle stretching and flexibility exercises, which can help improve joint mobility and reduce stiffness.

Enhanced Balance and Coordination: Certain movement-based meditations, such as Tai Chi or Qigong, focus on balance and coordination, which can help prevent falls and improve overall physical stability.

Pain Relief: Some forms of movement-based meditation, like yoga, can help alleviate chronic pain and improve posture, reducing discomfort and promoting physical well-being.

Stress Reduction: Movement-based meditation helps reduce stress and anxiety through mindful movement. The combination of physical activity and mindfulness techniques can release tension in the body and promote relaxation, which is particularly helpful for individuals who struggle with traditional seated meditation.

Improved Mind-Body Connection: Movement-based meditation encourages a deeper connection between the mind and body. By paying attention to bodily sensations, movement, and breath, practitioners become more attuned to their physical selves and can respond to stress and discomfort with greater awareness.

Enhanced Mindfulness: Engaging in mindful movement encourages practitioners to be fully present in the moment. This heightened state of mindfulness can lead to increased self-awareness and emotional regulation, which can be applied to daily life situations.

Accessible for Many Individuals: Movement-based meditation can be more accessible for people who find it challenging to sit still for extended periods or have physical limitations that make seated meditation uncomfortable. It offers an alternative approach to cultivating mindfulness.

Social and Community Aspect: Some movement-based meditation practices, like group yoga classes or dance meditation, provide opportunities for social interaction and community building. This can enhance the sense of belonging and support among practitioners.

Variety and Adaptability: There are numerous forms of movement-based meditation to choose from, such as yoga, Tai Chi, walking meditation, dance meditation, and more. This variety allows individuals to find a practice that suits their preferences and needs.

Enhanced Creativity: Movement-based meditation can stimulate creativity by encouraging a free flow of movement and expression. This can be especially beneficial for artists, writers, and individuals in creative professions.

Emotional Release: Some forms of movement-based meditation, like dance meditation, provide a safe space for emotional expression and release. Physical movement can help release pent-up emotions and promote emotional well-being.

Mindfulness Integration: The mindfulness skills developed in movement-based meditation can be integrated into daily life. Practitioners can apply these skills to reduce stress, enhance focus, and improve decision-making.

In summary, movement-based meditation offers a holistic approach to well-being by combining physical activity with mindfulness techniques. It can be particularly beneficial for those who struggle with traditional meditation methods or prefer a more dynamic practice. Ultimately, the advantages of movement-based meditation extend beyond physical health to encompass mental, emotional, and social well-being.

—————————————————

Yoga

Yoga is a comprehensive system of physical, mental, and spiritual practices that originated in ancient India. It has a rich history and has evolved over thousands of years into various forms and schools of thought. Yoga is not just a form of exercise but a holistic approach to achieving balance and harmony in one's life. Here are some key aspects to discuss about yoga:

Historical Background: Yoga dates back over 5,000 years to the Indus Valley Civilization. The earliest mention of yoga is found in the ancient Indian texts known as the Vedas. Over time, various yoga traditions and schools of thought have emerged, including Hatha, Bhakti, Jnana, Karma, and Kundalini yoga.

Physical Aspects: One of the most well-known aspects of yoga is the physical postures or asanas. Hatha yoga, for instance, focuses on these postures and is widely practiced in the West. These asanas help improve flexibility, strength, balance, and overall physical health.

Mental and Emotional Benefits: Yoga is also known for its profound impact on mental and emotional well-being. It incorporates mindfulness, meditation, and deep breathing techniques that can reduce stress, anxiety, and depression. Regular practice can improve mental clarity, concentration, and emotional stability.

Spiritual Connection: For many, yoga is a spiritual practice that fosters a deeper connection with oneself and the universe. It is often associated with Eastern philosophies and concepts like karma, dharma, and the chakras. Yoga can be a path to self-realization and enlightenment.

Different Yoga Styles: There are various styles of yoga, each with its own focus and emphasis. Some popular styles include:
    Hatha Yoga: Emphasizes physical postures and is great for

beginners.

Vinyasa Yoga: Focuses on breath and movement coordination, often in a flowing sequence.

Ashtanga Yoga: A rigorous and structured practice involving a specific sequence of poses.

Bikram Yoga: Performed in a hot room with a set sequence of 26 postures and two breathing exercises.

Iyengar Yoga: Emphasizes precision and alignment in poses, often using props.

Kundalini Yoga: A blend of postures, breathing exercises, and mantra chanting aimed at awakening spiritual energy.

Health Benefits: Yoga offers a wide range of health benefits, including improved flexibility, posture, and balance. It can also help alleviate chronic pain conditions, enhance cardiovascular health, and promote better sleep.

Mindfulness and Meditation: Yoga often includes practices in mindfulness and meditation, which have been scientifically proven to reduce stress, improve focus, and boost overall mental well-being.

Accessibility: Yoga is accessible to people of all ages and fitness levels. It can be modified to suit individual needs, making it inclusive and adaptable.

Yoga Philosophy: Beyond the physical postures, yoga encompasses a philosophical framework that encourages ethical behavior, self-discipline, and self-awareness.

Yoga in Modern Life: Yoga has become a global phenomenon, with millions of practitioners worldwide. It is used in various settings, including fitness studios, schools, workplaces, and even as a complementary therapy in healthcare.

In summary, yoga is a multifaceted practice that addresses physical, mental, and spiritual well-being. It has a rich history and continues to evolve to meet the needs of people seeking a holistic approach to health and self-awareness. Whether you are interested in physical fitness, stress reduction, or spiritual growth, yoga offers a versatile and comprehensive path to a balanced and harmonious life.

————————-

Tai Chi

Tai Chi, also spelled Taiji or Taijiquan, is a traditional Chinese martial art and mind-body practice that has gained popularity worldwide for its numerous health benefits and meditative qualities. It is often referred to as "moving meditation" due to its slow, flowing movements and emphasis on mindfulness. Tai Chi has a rich history and philosophy that encompasses physical, mental, and spiritual aspects. Here are some key aspects to discuss when it comes to Tai Chi:

History and Origins:

Tai Chi is believed to have been developed in China in the 17th century, attributed to a legendary figure named Zhang Sanfeng. It draws from ancient Chinese martial arts, Taoist philosophy, and traditional Chinese medicine. Over time, various styles and forms of Tai Chi have evolved, with the most well-known being the Yang, Chen, Wu, Sun, and Hao styles.

Principles and Philosophy:

Tai Chi is grounded in several fundamental principles, including:

Yin and Yang: Tai Chi seeks to balance the opposing forces of yin (softness) and yang (hardness) in both movement and life philosophy.

Qi (Chi): Central to Chinese philosophy, Tai Chi practitioners aim to cultivate and circulate the body's vital energy (Qi) through precise movements and breath control.

Centering: Maintaining a rooted center of balance is crucial in Tai Chi, promoting stability and fluidity in motion.

Movements and Forms:

Tai Chi consists of a series of choreographed movements or forms. These forms vary in complexity and can take anywhere from a few minutes to over an hour to complete. Movements are typically slow, graceful, and continuous, emphasizing precise postures, transitions, and controlled breathing. Beginners often start with shorter, simpler forms and progress to more advanced ones as they gain experience.

Health Benefits:

Tai Chi offers a wide range of physical and mental health benefits, including:

Improved Balance and Flexibility: Regular practice can enhance balance, flexibility, and coordination, making it particularly beneficial for older adults in preventing falls.

Stress Reduction: Tai Chi's meditative aspect can reduce stress and anxiety, promote relaxation, and improve mental well-being.

Enhanced Cardiovascular Health: While low-impact, Tai Chi can improve cardiovascular fitness, lower blood pressure, and reduce the risk of heart disease.

Pain Management: Some people find relief from chronic pain conditions like arthritis through Tai Chi practice.

Mindfulness: Tai Chi encourages mindfulness, helping practitioners become more aware of their bodies and thoughts.

Mind-Body Connection:

Tai Chi emphasizes the connection between mind and body. Practitioners focus on the present moment, maintain a relaxed state, and cultivate a deep awareness of their body's movements. This mind-body connection can lead to increased self-awareness and improved mental clarity.

Accessibility:

One of the great advantages of Tai Chi is its accessibility. It can be practiced by people of all ages and fitness levels. The slow and gentle nature of the movements makes it suitable for individuals with various physical limitations or health conditions.

Community and Cultural Significance:

Tai Chi is often practiced in groups or classes, fostering a sense of community and shared learning. It also plays a significant role in Chinese culture and traditional Chinese martial arts.

In summary, Tai Chi is a holistic practice that combines physical exercise, mental discipline, and philosophical principles. It offers a multitude of health benefits and can be a valuable addition to one's wellness routine, promoting both physical and mental well-being.

————————————

Walking Meditation

Walking meditation is a mindfulness practice that combines the physical act of walking with a meditative and present-focused mindset. It's a valuable alternative to traditional seated meditation for those who find it challenging to sit still for extended periods or prefer a more active approach to mindfulness. Walking meditation is often associated with various spiritual traditions, including Buddhism, but it can be practiced by people of all backgrounds and beliefs as a way to cultivate mindfulness, reduce stress, and enhance overall well-being.

Here are some key aspects and steps to practice walking meditation:

Choose a Quiet Location: Find a quiet and safe place to walk, such as a park, garden, or even a quiet room indoors. It should be an area where you can walk without interruptions or distractions.

Mindful Posture: Stand still for a moment and take a few deep breaths. Feel the weight of your body on your feet, and become aware of your posture. Stand up straight but not stiff, with your arms relaxed at your sides.

Start Walking Slowly: Begin to walk at a slow and deliberate pace. Pay close attention to each step you take. Notice the sensation of your foot lifting off the ground, moving through the air, and making contact with the earth. You can choose to walk in a straight line or in a small circle.

Focus on Your Breath: Coordinate your breath with your steps. For example, you might take one step with each inhale and one step with each exhale. This synchronizes your breathing with your movement, helping to anchor your awareness in the present moment.

Observe Sensations: As you walk, pay attention to the physical sensations in your body. Notice the feeling of the ground beneath your feet, the movement of your muscles, and any other bodily sensations that arise.

Stay Present: Your mind may wander, and that's normal. When you notice your thoughts drifting, gently bring your attention back to the act of walking. You can do this by focusing on your breath, the sensation of your feet, or the sounds around you.

Engage Your Senses: Explore your surroundings with your senses. Listen to the sounds of nature or the environment, feel the breeze or sun on your skin, and observe the colors and shapes around you.

Set an Intention: You can set an intention or focus for your walking meditation, such as cultivating gratitude, finding inner peace, or simply being present in the moment. This intention can guide your practice.

End Mindfully: When you're ready to conclude your walking meditation, slow down and come to a stop. Take a few moments to stand still and reflect on your experience. Notice how you feel mentally, emotionally, and physically.

Walking meditation can be adapted to different lengths of time, from a few minutes to longer sessions. It's a versatile practice that can be integrated into your daily routine, whether you're walking in a park, around your neighborhood, or even inside your home.

Ultimately, the goal of walking meditation is to cultivate mindfulness, reduce mental chatter, and increase your awareness of the present moment. Over time, this practice can lead to greater clarity, reduced stress, improved focus, and a deeper sense of connection with yourself and your surroundings.

––––––––––––––––––

Mantra and Affirmation Meditation

Mantra and affirmation meditation are two distinct approaches to meditation that involve the repetition of words, phrases, or sounds to achieve specific mental and spiritual benefits. While they share similarities in some aspects, they also have unique characteristics and purposes.

Mantra Meditation:

Mantra meditation is a traditional form of meditation that involves the repetition of a specific word, phrase, or sound known as a "mantra." Mantras can be a single word, a short phrase, or a series of syllables, and they are often chosen for their spiritual significance or vibrational qualities.

Purpose: The primary goal of mantra meditation is to quiet the mind and achieve a state of deep concentration or transcendence. It is a fundamental practice in various spiritual traditions, including Hinduism and Buddhism, and is believed to lead to spiritual growth and self-realization.

Technique: Practitioners typically sit comfortably with their eyes closed, silently repeating the chosen mantra. When distractions arise, they gently return their focus to the mantra. The repetition of the mantra helps to calm the mind and access deeper levels of consciousness.

Affirmation Meditation:

Affirmation meditation involves the repetition of positive affirmations or statements aimed at promoting self-improvement, self-confidence, and a positive mindset. Affirmations are often personalized and are intended to reinforce desired beliefs and attitudes.

Purpose: The main purpose of affirmation meditation is to reprogram the subconscious mind with positive beliefs and intentions. It is used as a tool for personal growth, building self-esteem, reducing stress, and achieving specific goals.

Technique: To practice affirmation meditation, individuals choose affirmations that resonate with their goals or intentions. They then repeat these affirmations either silently or aloud during meditation sessions. The goal is to ingrain these positive messages into the subconscious mind, which can influence thoughts, feelings, and behaviors.

Key Differences:

Focus: Mantra meditation focuses on achieving a state of deep concentration and inner stillness, while affirmation meditation emphasizes fostering positive beliefs and attitudes.

Content: Mantras are typically sacred words or sounds with spiritual significance, while affirmations are personalized, positive statements related to personal growth and well-being.

Goal: Mantra meditation often aims for spiritual enlightenment and self-realization, while affirmation meditation focuses on personal development and achieving specific life goals.

Traditions: Mantra meditation has deep roots in Hinduism and Buddhism, while affirmation meditation is a more modern practice rooted in self-help and personal development movements.

Both mantra and affirmation meditation can be valuable tools for self-improvement and mental well-being. The choice between the two depends on your goals and personal preferences. Some individuals may even integrate elements of both practices into their meditation routines to harness the benefits of both concentration and positive mindset cultivation.

————————————-

Choosing a mantra

Choosing a mantra is a personal and meaningful process that can have a profound impact on your meditation practice and overall well-being. A mantra is a word, phrase, or sound that is repeated during meditation to help focus the mind and achieve a state of inner peace and concentration. Here are some steps and considerations to help you choose the right mantra for you:

Understand the Purpose of a Mantra:

Mantras are used to calm the mind, reduce distractions, and deepen your meditation practice.

They can also have specific spiritual or personal significance, such as invoking positive qualities or intentions.

Reflect on Your Goals:

Consider your meditation goals. Are you looking for stress relief, inner peace, self-awareness, or spiritual growth?

Your chosen mantra should align with your intentions and aspirations.

Explore Different Types of Mantras:

There are various types of mantras, including religious or spiritual mantras, affirmations, and Sanskrit or sacred syllables.

You can choose a mantra from a particular tradition or create a personal mantra that resonates with you.

Traditional Mantras:

Traditional mantras often have deep cultural and spiritual significance. For example, "Om" is a universal and widely used mantra in Hinduism, Buddhism, and yoga.

Research different traditions and their associated mantras to find one that resonates with you.

Personal Affirmations:

Some people prefer to use personal affirmations as their mantra. These are positive statements that reflect your goals or values.

Examples include "I am at peace," "I am love," or "I am strong."

Test Different Mantras:

It's okay to experiment with different mantras to see which one feels most comfortable and effective for you.

Spend some time meditating with different mantras to gauge their impact on your state of mind and overall meditation experience.

Seek Guidance:

If you have a spiritual or meditation teacher, seek their guidance in choosing a mantra. They can offer insights based on your personal journey.

Some traditions require initiation or guidance from a qualified teacher for specific mantras.

Connect with the Sound or Meaning:

Choose a mantra that resonates with you on a deep level, whether through its sound, meaning, or symbolism.

The mantra should evoke a sense of calm, focus, or spirituality when you repeat it.

Commitment and Consistency:

Once you choose a mantra, commit to using it consistently in your meditation practice.

Repetition is key to experiencing the full benefits of a mantra.

Adapt Over Time:

As your meditation practice evolves and your goals change, be open to reevaluating and possibly changing your mantra.

Mantras can evolve with you as you grow and develop on your spiritual journey.

Remember that the process of choosing a mantra is highly

individual. There is no one-size-fits-all approach, so trust your intuition and choose a mantra that resonates with your heart and mind. With dedication and practice, your chosen mantra can become a powerful tool for inner transformation and self-discovery.

————————————————-

Positive affirmations for focus

Positive affirmations are statements or phrases that you repeat to yourself regularly to help shift your mindset in a positive direction. When it comes to focus, affirmations can be a powerful tool to boost your concentration, productivity, and overall mental clarity. Here are some positive affirmations for focus:

"I am fully present in this moment."

This affirmation reminds you to stay in the present and not get distracted by past regrets or future worries.

"My mind is sharp and alert."

Repeating this affirmation can help you feel mentally prepared and capable of tackling tasks that require focus.

"I easily maintain my concentration on the task at hand."

Use this affirmation to reinforce your ability to stay focused and avoid distractions.

"I am in control of my thoughts and actions."

This affirmation empowers you to take charge of your mind

and direct your attention where it needs to be.

"I am disciplined and dedicated to achieving my goals."
By repeating this affirmation, you reaffirm your commitment to staying focused on your long-term objectives.

"I find joy and satisfaction in my work."
Focusing on the positive aspects of your tasks can help you stay engaged and attentive.

"I embrace challenges as opportunities to grow."
This affirmation can shift your perspective on difficult tasks, making them seem less daunting and more engaging.

"I prioritize my tasks and manage my time effectively."
Remind yourself of your time management skills to help you allocate your focus where it's needed most.

"I am in tune with my intuition and make sound decisions."
Trusting your instincts can enhance your ability to concentrate on the choices you make.

"I release all thoughts that do not serve my current goals."
Use this affirmation to let go of distracting or negative thoughts that hinder your focus.

"I am patient and persistent in my pursuit of success."
Patience can help you maintain your focus over the long term, especially when facing challenges.

"I am fully engaged in the present task, and I am making

progress."

This affirmation reinforces your commitment to the task at hand and acknowledges your achievements, no matter how small.

"I am grateful for my ability to concentrate and be productive."

Expressing gratitude for your focus can help you appreciate and nurture this valuable skill.

Remember that affirmations are most effective when repeated regularly and with genuine belief. You can incorporate these affirmations into your daily routine, such as reciting them in the morning, during breaks, or whenever you need a boost of focus and motivation. Over time, these positive affirmations can help you strengthen your ability to stay focused on your goals and tasks.

———————————————

Strategies for digital detox

Digital detox refers to the practice of temporarily reducing or eliminating your use of digital devices and online activities to promote mental and physical well-being. In today's hyper-connected world, where we are constantly bombarded with notifications and information, a digital detox can be a valuable strategy to regain focus, reduce stress, and reconnect with the real world. Here are some strategies for a successful digital detox:

Set clear goals:

Define the purpose of your digital detox. Are you looking

to reduce screen time, improve sleep, boost productivity, or simply find more time for offline activities? Having a clear goal will help you stay motivated.

Establish boundaries:

Create specific rules and guidelines for your digital detox. For example, you might decide to limit screen time to a certain number of hours per day or designate specific times when you'll be completely offline.

Notify others:

Let your friends, family, and colleagues know about your digital detox plans. Informing them in advance will help manage expectations and reduce the pressure to respond to messages or emails promptly.

Turn off notifications:

Disable non-essential notifications on your devices to reduce distractions. You can choose to receive notifications only for essential communication apps and mute or turn off others.

Designate tech-free zones:

Designate certain areas of your home or specific times of day as tech-free zones or periods. This can help you disconnect from screens and engage in offline activities without temptation.

Unplug gradually:

If going completely offline is too challenging, consider a gradual approach. Start by reducing your screen time incrementally until you reach your desired level of digital detox.

Find offline alternatives:

Identify activities you enjoy doing offline, such as reading, exercising, cooking, or spending time with friends and family. Engaging in these activities can help fill the void left by digital devices.

Use digital tools mindfully:

When you do use digital devices, practice mindful consumption. Be selective about the content you engage with and avoid mindless scrolling. Set time limits for specific apps or websites.

Delete unnecessary apps:

Review your smartphone or tablet and delete apps that don't serve a meaningful purpose or contribute to your digital detox goals. This can reduce the temptation to use them.

Consider a digital detox app:

There are apps available that can help you track your screen time and set usage limits. Some even lock you out of certain apps or websites during designated times.

Replace screens with physical activities:

Physical activities like walking, jogging, or practicing yoga can be excellent substitutes for screen time. They promote better health and well-being.

Practice self-awareness:

Pay attention to your digital habits and how they make you feel. Reflect on the positive changes you experience during your digital detox to reinforce the habit.

Seek support:

Consider involving friends or family members in your digital detox journey. They can provide encouragement and accountability.

Evaluate and adjust:

Periodically review your digital detox progress and adjust your strategies as needed. You may find that certain aspects of your plan are more effective than others.

Remember that a digital detox doesn't have to be a complete break from technology; it can be tailored to your needs and lifestyle. The key is to find a balance that allows you to enjoy the benefits of technology without being overwhelmed by it.

––––––––––––

Mindful screen time

Mindful screen time refers to the practice of using digital devices and engaging with digital content in a conscious and intentional way, with a focus on promoting mental and emotional well-being. In today's digital age, where screens are an integral part of our daily lives, practicing mindful screen time has become increasingly important to strike a balance between technology use and maintaining a healthy lifestyle. Here are some key aspects of mindful screen time:

Awareness: Mindful screen time begins with self-awareness. It involves recognizing and acknowledging your digital habits, such as how much time you spend on screens, which apps or websites you use most frequently, and how these habits affect your well-being.

Set Boundaries: Once you are aware of your digital habits, you can set boundaries for screen time. This might include allocating specific time slots for device use and sticking to those limits. For example, you could establish "no-screen" zones or times during meals, before bedtime, or when spending quality time with family and friends.

Quality over Quantity: Instead of mindlessly scrolling through social media or watching endless cat videos, practice using screens for meaningful and purposeful activities. Engage in activities that promote learning, creativity, and personal growth.

Digital Detox: Periodically disconnecting from screens can be rejuvenating. Consider taking a digital detox weekend or a screen-free day to recharge and reconnect with the physical world. This break allows you to reset your relationship with screens.

Single-Tasking: Multitasking on screens often leads to decreased productivity and increased stress. Try to focus on one task at a time, whether it's work-related, reading, or leisure activities. Mindful screen time encourages single-tasking to enhance concentration and reduce stress.

Mindful Consumption: Be conscious of the content you consume. Avoid mindless scrolling through news feeds and instead seek out content that is informative, inspiring, or entertaining in a positive way. Unfollow or mute accounts that consistently make you feel negative emotions.

Digital Well-Being Tools: Many devices and apps now include features to help you manage your screen time. These tools can help you track your usage, set app limits, and even remind you to take breaks.

Prioritize Real-Life Connections: While screens can facilitate connections, don't forget to prioritize face-to-face interactions with friends and family. Maintain a healthy balance between digital and real-life relationships.

Practice Mindfulness: Incorporate mindfulness techniques into your digital routine. This can include taking a few deep breaths before checking your phone, being fully present when engaging in digital activities, and regularly checking in with your emotions and stress levels.

Evaluate and Adjust: Regularly evaluate your mindful screen time practices and make adjustments as needed. Your needs and circumstances may change, so it's essential to remain flexible and adapt your screen time habits accordingly.

Incorporating these principles of mindful screen time into your daily life can help you maintain a healthy relationship with technology and promote your overall well-being. Remember that the goal is not to eliminate screen time entirely but to use screens in a way that enhances your life without detracting from it.

Five

Overcoming Common Challenges

Strategies for calming a busy mind:

Dealing with Restlessness

Calming a busy mind is essential for mental well-being and can improve focus, reduce stress, and enhance overall quality of life. Here are some effective strategies to help you calm a busy mind:

Meditation and Mindfulness:

Regular meditation practice can help you become more aware of your thoughts and emotions and create a sense of inner peace.

Mindfulness techniques, such as deep breathing and body scans, can ground you in the present moment and reduce racing thoughts.

Deep Breathing Exercises:

Deep, slow breaths can trigger the body's relaxation response. Try inhaling deeply through your nose for a count of four, holding for four, and exhaling slowly through your mouth for a count of four.

Progressive Muscle Relaxation:

This technique involves tensing and then relaxing each muscle group in your body, starting from your toes and moving up to your head. It can help release physical tension and calm your mind.

Yoga:

Yoga combines physical postures with breathing exercises and meditation. It promotes relaxation and can help reduce stress and anxiety.

Journaling:

Writing down your thoughts and feelings can help you process and make sense of them. It can also provide a sense of relief and closure.

Nature and Fresh Air:

Spending time in nature or simply getting fresh air can be incredibly soothing. Take a walk in a park or sit outside for a few minutes to clear your mind.

Limit Stimulants:

Reduce or eliminate the consumption of caffeine, nicotine, and other stimulants, especially in the evening, as they can contribute to a busy mind and disrupt sleep.

Establish a Routine:

Creating a daily schedule can help reduce mental clutter. Knowing what to expect and when can create a sense of order and calm.

Prioritize and Organize:

Break tasks into smaller, manageable steps, and prioritize them. This can prevent overwhelm and reduce racing thoughts about all you have to do.

Digital Detox:

Take breaks from screens and social media. Constant notifications and information overload can contribute to a busy mind.

Progressive Relaxation Techniques:

Engage in activities like progressive muscle relaxation or autogenic training to systematically relax your body and mind.

Guided Imagery and Visualization:

Listen to or practice guided imagery exercises that take you to calming and serene mental landscapes. This can help shift your focus away from racing thoughts.

Limit Multitasking:

Focus on one task at a time rather than trying to do several things simultaneously. Multitasking can overwhelm your mind and reduce productivity.

Seek Professional Help:

If your busy mind is accompanied by excessive stress, anxiety, or other mental health concerns, consider speaking with a therapist or counselor who can provide guidance and support.

Mindful Movement:
Engage in activities like tai chi or qigong, which combine gentle movements with mindfulness to promote relaxation.

Affirmations and Positive Self-talk:
Use positive affirmations to challenge and replace negative or racing thoughts with more calming and constructive ones.

Remember that finding the right combination of strategies may take some experimentation, and it's okay to adapt your approach over time as your needs change. Consistency and patience are key when it comes to calming a busy mind.

Embracing imperfections in meditation

Embracing imperfections in meditation is an important aspect of developing a sustainable and fulfilling meditation practice. Meditation is not about achieving perfection but rather about cultivating mindfulness, self-compassion, and personal growth. Here are some key points to consider when it comes to embracing imperfections in meditation:

Understanding Imperfection: Recognize that imperfection is a fundamental aspect of being human. Everyone experiences distractions, wandering thoughts, restlessness, and physical discomfort during meditation. These imperfections are not failures but natural parts of the meditation process.

Non-Judgmental Awareness: Meditation encourages non-judgmental awareness. When you notice imperfections or distractions during your practice, try to observe them without judgment. Instead of labeling your experience as good or bad, simply acknowledge what is happening without attachment.

Self-Compassion: Embrace imperfections with self-compassion. Treat yourself with the same kindness and understanding that you would offer to a friend. Remember that it's okay to have a wandering mind or to feel restless; these are opportunities for growth, not reasons for self-criticism.

Gentle Redirecting: When you notice your mind wandering or getting caught up in imperfections, gently redirect your focus back to your chosen point of meditation, whether it's your breath, a mantra, or another anchor. This redirection is a crucial skill in meditation, and it's something you can practice and refine over time.

Consistency over Perfection: Consistency in your meditation practice is more important than perfection in any individual session. The cumulative benefits of regular meditation come from a long-term commitment to the practice, not from having flawless sessions every time.

Mindful Growth: Imperfections in meditation can be seen as opportunities for growth and self-awareness. They reveal areas where your mind might need more training or where you can explore deeper aspects of your consciousness. Every moment of meditation, even imperfect ones, contributes to your personal development.

Adjust Expectations: Adjust your expectations about meditation. Instead of aiming for a perfect, distraction-free experience, focus on simply being present in the moment. Over time, you may notice improvements in your ability to sustain your attention, but this will come with practice and patience.

Seek Guidance: If you find it challenging to embrace imperfections in your meditation practice, consider seeking guidance from a meditation teacher or a meditation group. They can offer insights, techniques, and support to help you navigate these challenges.

In summary, embracing imperfections in meditation is an integral part of the practice. It's through the acknowledgment and acceptance of these imperfections that you can truly grow and benefit from meditation. Remember that meditation is a journey, not a destination, and it's okay to be imperfect along the way. It's in those imperfect moments that you have the opportunity to cultivate mindfulness, self-compassion, and a deeper understanding of yourself.

———————————————

Handling Impatience

Impatience is a common human emotion characterized by a strong desire for something to happen quickly or without delay. It often arises when individuals are faced with situations that require waiting, and they find the waiting process frustrating or intolerable. Impatience can manifest in various aspects of life, from small everyday inconveniences to more significant long-term goals, and it can have both positive and negative consequences.

Here are some key aspects of impatience to consider:

Causes of Impatience:
Instant Gratification Culture: In today's fast-paced world, people have grown accustomed to instant access to information, services, and products. This culture of instant gratification can lead to impatience when things don't happen quickly.
Time Pressure: Tight schedules and deadlines can make people more prone to impatience, as they feel the pressure to get things done quickly.
Uncertainty: Not knowing when or how something will happen can trigger impatience, as people seek certainty and control over their circumstances.
Personal Expectations: Unrealistic expectations about how quickly a task or goal should be achieved can contribute to impatience when those expectations aren't met.

Positive Aspects of Impatience:
Drive and Motivation: Impatience can serve as a motivator, pushing individuals to work harder and more efficiently to achieve their goals sooner.
Problem-Solving: Impatience can lead to creative problem-solving when individuals are eager to overcome obstacles and find quicker solutions.
Productivity: In some cases, impatience can increase productivity, as people may try to accomplish tasks more rapidly to reduce their frustration.

Negative Aspects of Impatience:

Stress and Anxiety: Frequent impatience can lead to chronic stress and anxiety, as individuals are often on edge and unable to relax.

Impulsivity: Impatience can lead to impulsive decision-making, where individuals make hasty choices without considering the consequences.

Relationship Strain: Impatience can strain relationships, as it can lead to irritability and impatience with others' perceived slowness or inefficiency.

Strategies to Manage Impatience:

Mindfulness and Relaxation Techniques: Practicing mindfulness, meditation, or deep breathing exercises can help individuals stay calm and reduce feelings of impatience.

Setting Realistic Expectations: Adjusting expectations to align with the actual timeframes required for tasks or goals can reduce impatience.

Time Management: Effective time management skills can help individuals allocate their time more efficiently and reduce the pressure that leads to impatience.

Communication: Open and honest communication with others can help manage impatience in relationships by setting clear expectations and addressing concerns.

Cultural and Societal Influences: Impatience can vary across cultures and societies. Some cultures place a higher value on patience, while others prioritize speed and efficiency. These cultural norms can influence how individuals perceive and manage impatience.

In conclusion, impatience is a complex emotion that arises

from various factors, including societal pressures and personal expectations. While it can have both positive and negative effects, understanding and managing impatience is important for maintaining mental and emotional well-being, as well as for achieving long-term goals and maintaining healthy relationships.

––––––––––––––––––––––––––––––-

Cultivating patience through practice

Cultivating patience through practice is a valuable skill that can lead to personal growth, improved relationships, and enhanced well-being. Patience is the ability to endure difficult situations or delays without becoming frustrated, and it's a quality that can be developed and honed over time. Here are some key aspects of how to cultivate patience through practice:

Mindfulness Meditation: Mindfulness meditation is a practice that encourages you to be present in the moment without judgment. By regularly meditating, you can become more aware of your thoughts, emotions, and reactions. This awareness allows you to better understand your impatience and learn to manage it effectively.

Set Realistic Expectations: Impatience often arises when we set unrealistic expectations for ourselves or others. Practice setting realistic goals and timelines. This will reduce the likelihood of disappointment and frustration when things don't go as planned.

Practice Delayed Gratification: Delayed gratification involves intentionally delaying immediate rewards for long-term benefits. Start small, like delaying your consumption of a favorite snack or postponing a purchase. Gradually, you can apply this principle to more significant aspects of your life, such as saving money or pursuing long-term goals.

Deep Breathing and Relaxation Techniques: When you feel impatience building, practice deep breathing and relaxation techniques. Deep, slow breaths can help calm your nervous system and reduce stress, making it easier to remain patient in challenging situations.

Mindful Communication: In your interactions with others, practice mindful communication. Listen actively and without interruption, and respond thoughtfully instead of reacting impulsively. This can lead to better understanding and more constructive conversations, reducing impatience and frustration in relationships.

Learn from Mistakes: Patience often requires the ability to learn from mistakes and setbacks. Instead of dwelling on your failures, view them as opportunities for growth. By practicing resilience and persistence, you'll develop greater patience in the face of adversity.

Practice Gratitude: Cultivating gratitude can help you appreciate the present moment and reduce the desire for instant gratification. Regularly reflect on the things you are grateful for, which can shift your focus away from impatience.

Engage in Patience-Building Activities: Engage in activities that inherently require patience, such as puzzles, gardening, or learning a musical instrument. These activities can help you develop perseverance and tolerance for delayed rewards.

Seek Role Models: Identify individuals in your life or in the public sphere who exemplify patience. Study their behavior, how they handle difficult situations, and their ability to remain calm and composed. Learn from their examples and apply their strategies in your life.

Track Your Progress: Keep a journal to track your progress in developing patience. Record situations where you've successfully exercised patience and those where you struggled. Reflect on what worked and what didn't, and use this information to refine your practice.

Remember that cultivating patience is an ongoing process, and setbacks are natural. Be patient with yourself as you work to develop this skill, and acknowledge that it may take time to see significant changes. With consistent practice and dedication, you can enhance your patience, leading to a more peaceful and resilient life. Be sure to set realistic expectations – remember to take baby steps!

——————————————————

Building a consistent meditation routine

Building a consistent meditation routine is crucial for various reasons, as it can have a profound and lasting impact on your physical, mental, and emotional well-being. Here are some key reasons why consistency in meditation practice is essential:

Stress Reduction: Meditation is a powerful tool for managing stress. When you meditate regularly, you train your mind to become more resilient to stressors. Consistency helps you develop the skills to remain calm and composed in challenging situations, reducing the harmful effects of chronic stress on your body and mind.

Improved Focus and Concentration: Meditation enhances your ability to concentrate and stay focused. Regular practice strengthens your attention muscles, making it easier to concentrate on tasks, problem-solving, and decision-making in your daily life.

Emotional Regulation: Meditation helps you become more aware of your emotions and how to respond to them in a balanced way. Consistent practice can reduce emotional reactivity, allowing you to handle difficult emotions like anger, anxiety, and sadness more skillfully.

Mindfulness: Building a consistent meditation routine is an effective way to cultivate mindfulness. Mindfulness involves being fully present in the moment, without judgment. Regular meditation practice deepens your capacity for mindfulness, which can lead to greater self-awareness and a richer experience of life.

Enhanced Well-being: Meditation has been linked to increased feelings of happiness, contentment, and overall well-being. A consistent practice can help you develop a more positive outlook on life and a greater sense of inner peace.

Better Sleep: Many people struggle with sleep issues, and meditation can be a natural remedy. Regular meditation can improve sleep quality by reducing racing thoughts and promoting relaxation.

Physical Health Benefits: Meditation has been associated with various physical health benefits, such as lowered blood pressure, improved immune function, and reduced inflammation. Consistency is key to reaping these long-term health rewards.

Personal Growth and Self-Discovery: Meditation can be a journey of self-discovery. Over time, you may gain insights into your thought patterns, habits, and beliefs. Consistency allows you to explore these aspects of yourself more deeply and make positive changes as needed.

Neuroplasticity: Meditation can actually change the structure and function of your brain through a process called neuroplasticity. Consistent practice can lead to the development of new neural pathways associated with greater emotional resilience and cognitive flexibility.

Spiritual Growth: For those on a spiritual path, meditation can deepen their connection to their inner self or higher power. Consistency in practice often leads to profound spiritual insights and experiences.

To build and maintain a consistent meditation routine, it's essential to start small and gradually increase your practice time as you become more comfortable. Finding a time and place that works for you, setting realistic goals, and using guided meditations or apps can also help you establish a routine.

Remember that the benefits of meditation typically accrue over time, so patience and commitment are essential. By incorporating meditation into your daily life and making it a habit, you can experience significant and lasting improvements in your overall well-being.

———————————————-

Navigating Inner Resistance - Understanding resistance to change

Understanding resistance to change in the context of meditation can be a valuable aspect of personal growth and self-awareness. Change, even when it's positive, can evoke resistance because it often challenges our established habits and beliefs. Here's how you can explore and address resistance to change in meditation:

Awareness: Begin by cultivating mindfulness during your meditation practice. Pay close attention to your thoughts, emotions, and bodily sensations. As you meditate, you may notice resistance manifesting as restlessness, discomfort, or a strong urge to stop meditating.

Self-Inquiry: Ask yourself why you're experiencing resistance. Is it because you're trying a new meditation technique or sitting for a longer duration? Are you encountering uncomfortable emotions or thoughts? Understanding the root cause of your resistance is essential for addressing it.

Acceptance: In meditation, as in life, it's crucial to practice acceptance. Acknowledge your resistance without judgment. Understand that resistance is a natural reaction to change and doesn't make you inadequate or incapable of meditating effectively.

Explore Beliefs: Resistance often stems from beliefs and expectations. Examine your beliefs about meditation. Are you expecting instant results or a completely tranquil mind? Such expectations can lead to resistance when they aren't met. Adjust your expectations to be more realistic.

Gentle Persistence: Instead of trying to force yourself to meditate, approach it with gentleness and persistence. If resistance arises, don't fight it. Continue with your meditation practice, even if it means sitting with uncomfortable feelings. Over time, this persistence can help reduce resistance.

Gradual Progression: If you're making significant changes to your meditation practice, consider a gradual approach. Incrementally increase the duration of your sessions or explore different techniques step by step. This can make change feel less overwhelming.

Seek Guidance: If you're struggling with resistance to change in your meditation practice, consider seeking guidance from an experienced meditation teacher or therapist. They can provide personalized insights and techniques to help you navigate resistance.

Journaling: Keeping a meditation journal can be beneficial. Write down your experiences, including any resistance you encounter. Reflect on these entries to gain deeper insights into your patterns of resistance and how they relate to your life outside of meditation.

Group Support: Joining a meditation group or community can offer valuable support. Sharing your experiences and challenges with others who are on a similar path can help you feel less alone in your struggles with resistance.

Celebrate Progress: Celebrate small victories along your meditation journey. When you successfully navigate resistance and experience moments of clarity, peace, or insight, acknowledge and celebrate these moments. Positive reinforcement can motivate you to continue embracing change.

Understanding resistance to change in meditation is an essential aspect of personal growth and self-awareness. By approaching it with mindfulness, self-inquiry, and patience, you can gradually overcome resistance and experience the transformative benefits of meditation in your life.

— — — — — — — — — — — — — — — -

Overcoming self-sabotage

Overcoming self-sabotage is a crucial step towards personal growth, achieving goals, and leading a fulfilling life. Self-sabotage refers to behaviors, thoughts, or actions that undermine your own success or well-being. It can manifest in various forms, such as procrastination, self-doubt, perfectionism, fear of failure, or negative self-talk. Recognizing and addressing self-sabotage is essential for achieving your full potential. Here are some strategies to help you overcome self-sabotage:

Self-awareness: The first step in overcoming self-sabotage is to become aware of it. Pay attention to your thoughts, emotions, and behaviors to identify patterns of self-sabotaging tendencies. Keep a journal to track these patterns and gain insight into what triggers them.

Understand the root causes: Self-sabotage often has deep-rooted causes, such as past traumas, limiting beliefs, or fear of success. Take time to reflect on the underlying reasons for your self-sabotaging behavior. Therapy or counseling can be beneficial in exploring these issues with a professional.

Set clear goals: Establishing clear and achievable goals can provide you with direction and motivation. When you have a purpose and a plan, it becomes easier to resist self-sabotaging behaviors that derail your progress.

Challenge limiting beliefs: Identify and challenge any negative beliefs you have about yourself, your abilities, or your worthiness of success. Replace these beliefs with more empowering and positive affirmations.

Cultivate self-compassion: Be kind and gentle with yourself, especially when you make mistakes or encounter setbacks. Self-criticism can fuel self-sabotage, so practice self-compassion and treat yourself with the same kindness you would offer to a friend.

Break tasks into smaller steps: Overwhelming tasks can lead to procrastination and self-sabotage. Break down your goals into smaller, manageable steps, making it easier to take action and build momentum.

Develop a support system: Share your goals and struggles with supportive friends, family members, or a mentor. Having a support system can provide accountability, encouragement, and guidance when you need it.

Practice mindfulness: Mindfulness techniques, such as meditation and deep breathing exercises, can help you become more aware of your thoughts and emotions in the moment. This awareness can help you interrupt self-sabotaging thought patterns and make more constructive choices.

Develop resilience: Understand that setbacks and failures are a natural part of life. Embrace them as opportunities for growth rather than as evidence of your inadequacy. Resilience can help you bounce back from setbacks and continue working towards your goals.

Seek professional help: If self-sabotage is significantly impacting your life, consider working with a therapist or counselor who specializes in self-sabotage or related issues. They can provide tailored strategies and support to help you overcome these challenges.

Overcoming self-sabotage is a gradual process that requires patience and persistence. It's essential to remember that setbacks are normal, and you may still experience moments of self-sabotage along the way. However, with self-awareness and a commitment to personal growth, you can gradually reduce self-sabotaging behaviors and create a more positive and fulfilling life.

Integrating Meditation into Daily Life

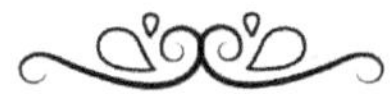

Mindful Eating

Mindful eating is a practice that encourages individuals to develop a more conscious and attentive relationship with their food. It's rooted in the principles of mindfulness, a meditation technique that involves paying purposeful attention to the present moment without judgment. The idea behind mindful eating is to bring the same level of mindfulness to the act of eating as one would to meditation. Here are some key aspects and benefits of mindful eating:

Awareness of Sensations: Mindful eating involves paying close attention to the sensory aspects of eating, such as the taste, smell, texture, and even the sounds of the food. This heightened awareness can enhance the overall eating experience and make it more enjoyable.

Slower Eating: Mindful eating encourages a slower pace of eating. By savoring each bite and chewing food thoroughly, individuals become more in tune with their body's hunger and fullness cues. This can help prevent overeating and promote a healthier relationship with food.

Eating with Intention: Instead of mindlessly consuming food out of habit or boredom, mindful eating encourages individuals to eat with intention. Before eating, take a moment to consider why you're eating and whether you're genuinely hungry or simply seeking comfort or distraction.

Elimination of Distractions: Many people eat while multi-tasking, such as watching TV, working, or scrolling through their phones. Mindful eating suggests removing distractions and focusing solely on the act of eating, which can lead to better portion control and increased enjoyment of meals.

Recognition of Emotional Eating: Mindful eating helps individuals recognize emotional triggers that lead to unhealthy eating habits. By becoming aware of the emotions driving their food choices, individuals can develop healthier coping mechanisms for dealing with stress, sadness, or other emotions.

Listening to Hunger and Fullness Signals: Paying attention to physical hunger and fullness cues is a central aspect of mindful eating. This can help individuals stop eating when they are satisfied rather than continuing to eat based on external factors like portion size or social pressure. Keep in mind, however, that these signals may not occur immediately, especially as one gets older.

Improved Digestion: Eating mindfully may improve digestion by allowing the body to better process and absorb nutrients. Chewing food thoroughly, for example, aids in the initial breakdown of food, which can make digestion more efficient.

Weight Management: Some studies suggest that practicing mindful eating can aid in weight management. By reducing overeating and promoting healthier food choices, individuals may naturally achieve and maintain a healthier weight.

Reduced Stress: Mindful eating can be a form of stress reduction. Taking time to enjoy a meal in a relaxed and focused manner can help individuals feel calmer and more centered.

Enhanced Gratitude: Mindful eating encourages gratitude for the food we have and the effort that goes into producing it. This gratitude can foster a greater connection with the food we consume and a deeper appreciation for the nourishment it provides.

To start practicing mindful eating, you can begin by setting aside dedicated meal times free from distractions, focusing on the sensory experience of eating, and paying attention to your body's hunger and fullness cues. Over time, with practice, mindful eating can become a natural and more fulfilling way to approach meals, leading to a healthier and more balanced relationship with food.

————————

Mindful Communication

Mindful communication refers to the practice of being fully present and attentive when engaging in conversations with others. It involves active listening, empathy, and conscious awareness of your words and actions. This approach to communication offers a wide range of benefits in personal and professional settings:

Improved Understanding: Mindful communication helps you better understand the thoughts, feelings, and perspectives of others. By actively listening without judgment, you can gain deeper insights into their needs and concerns.

Enhanced Relationships: Mindful communication fosters stronger and more positive relationships. When people feel heard and respected, they are more likely to trust and connect with you on a deeper level.

Conflict Resolution: Mindfulness can be a powerful tool in resolving conflicts. By staying calm and present during difficult conversations, you can avoid escalating conflicts and work towards finding mutually satisfactory solutions.

Reduced Stress: Mindful communication can reduce stress and anxiety in both the speaker and the listener. When you approach conversations with a sense of mindfulness, you are less likely to react impulsively or defensively, leading to more relaxed interactions.

Increased Empathy: Mindfulness encourages empathy by encouraging you to put yourself in the other person's shoes. This can lead to greater understanding and compassion, which is especially valuable in sensitive or emotionally charged conversations.

Better Decision-Making: Mindful communication helps you make more informed decisions. By carefully considering the information shared in a conversation, you are less likely to make hasty judgments or decisions based on incomplete information.

Enhanced Self-Awareness: Practicing mindful communication can also increase your self-awareness. When you pay attention to your thoughts, emotions, and communication patterns, you can identify areas for personal growth and development.

Improved Listening Skills: Mindful communication involves active listening, which means you are fully engaged in the conversation rather than just waiting for your turn to speak. This improves your ability to absorb information and respond thoughtfully.

Better Communication Outcomes: Mindfulness can lead to more effective communication outcomes. When you are fully present in a conversation, you are more likely to convey your message clearly and ensure that it is understood as intended.

Personal Growth: Mindful communication is a continuous

practice that encourages personal growth. It can help you become a more patient, empathetic, and compassionate individual, which can positively impact all areas of your life.

Professional Advantages: In a professional context, mindful communication can lead to better teamwork, increased productivity, and improved leadership skills. It can also be an asset in negotiation and conflict resolution.

Health Benefits: Research has shown that practicing mindfulness, including mindful communication, can have physical and psychological health benefits. It can reduce stress, improve emotional well-being, and even boost the immune system.

In summary, mindful communication offers a wide range of benefits, including improved understanding, stronger relationships, better conflict resolution, reduced stress, increased empathy, and personal growth. By incorporating mindfulness into your communication style, you can enhance both your personal and professional interactions.

––––––––––––

Active listening techniques

Active listening is a fundamental communication skill that involves not just hearing words but also understanding, interpreting, and responding to what someone is saying in a thoughtful and engaged manner. It's a crucial skill in various personal and professional contexts, such as relationships, conflict resolution, customer service, and leadership. Here are some key techniques and strategies for active listening:

Give your full attention: Make a conscious effort to focus solely on the speaker and eliminate distractions. Put away your phone, close your laptop, and give them your undivided attention.

Maintain eye contact: Establishing and maintaining eye contact demonstrates that you are engaged and attentive. However, be mindful not to make the other person uncomfortable by staring.

Show empathy: Try to understand the speaker's perspective and feelings. Show empathy by nodding, using facial expressions that convey understanding, and providing verbal cues like "I see," "I understand," or "That must have been difficult."

Avoid interrupting: Resist the urge to interrupt or interject your thoughts while the speaker is talking. Let them finish their point before you respond.

Use nonverbal cues: Nonverbal cues, such as body language and facial expressions, can convey your interest and understanding. Leaning slightly forward, mirroring the speaker's body language (in a non-awkward way), and nodding can be effective nonverbal signals.

Paraphrase and summarize: Periodically repeat back what you've heard to confirm your understanding and show that you're actively processing the information. Phrases like "So, if I understand correctly, you're saying..." can be helpful.

Ask open-ended questions: Encourage the speaker to share more by asking open-ended questions that require more than a simple yes or no answer. For example, "Can you tell me more about that?" or "How did that make you feel?"

Reflect feelings: Reflecting the speaker's emotions can help them feel heard and validated. You might say, "It sounds like you're really frustrated about this situation."

Avoid judgment and assumptions: Suspend judgment and refrain from making assumptions or jumping to conclusions about the speaker's words or intentions. Stay open-minded and objective.

Provide feedback: Offer constructive feedback and responses that show you are actively engaged in the conversation. Share your thoughts and opinions when appropriate, but do so in a way that respects the speaker's perspective.

Be patient: Sometimes, people need time to gather their thoughts or express themselves fully. Be patient and give them the space they need.

Manage your own emotions: Stay emotionally balanced and avoid becoming defensive or confrontational, especially if the conversation involves sensitive or difficult topics.

Practice silence: Don't feel the need to fill every moment with words. Silence can be powerful and give the speaker space to collect their thoughts and continue speaking.

Active listening is a skill that can be developed and refined with practice. It not only helps you better understand others but also strengthens relationships and promotes effective communication.

Mindful speaking and empathy

Mindful speaking and empathy are two interconnected concepts that play a crucial role in effective communication and building strong, positive relationships. Let's delve into each of these concepts and explore how they relate to each other:

Mindful Speaking: Mindful speaking, also known as mindful communication, is a practice rooted in mindfulness, which involves being fully present and conscious in the way you express yourself verbally. It emphasizes awareness, intentionality, and authenticity in your words and interactions. Here are some key principles of mindful speaking:

Presence: Mindful speaking begins with being fully present in the moment and paying close attention to the conversation without distractions or preconceived judgments. This presence allows you to engage more deeply with the other person.

Self-awareness: Before speaking, it's important to reflect on your thoughts, emotions, and intentions. This self-awareness helps you choose your words more consciously and avoid impulsive or harmful remarks.

Non-judgment: Mindful speaking encourages non-judgmental listening and speaking. It means refraining from making assumptions, labeling, or criticizing the other person's perspectives or feelings.

Kindness and compassion: Approach conversations with an open heart and a desire to connect with others on a human level. Use language that is considerate, respectful, and empathetic.

Clarity and brevity: Strive for clear and concise communication to ensure your message is easily understood. Avoid unnecessary jargon, rambling, or vague language.

Empathy: Empathy is the ability to understand and share the feelings and perspectives of others. It involves stepping into someone else's shoes, seeing the world from their point of view, and responding with compassion. Empathy plays a crucial role in building meaningful relationships and fostering emotional connections. Here are some aspects of empathy:

Active listening: Empathy starts with active listening, which means giving your full attention to the speaker, making eye contact, and showing that you are genuinely interested in what they have to say. This helps create a safe space for them to express themselves.

Perspective-taking: Try to understand the other person's thoughts, feelings, and experiences from their perspective. This requires setting aside your own judgments and biases.

Validation: Empathetic communication involves acknowledging and validating the other person's emotions, even if you don't necessarily agree with their point of view. Validation helps people feel heard and understood.

Emotional support: When someone is going through a tough time, empathy involves offering emotional support and comfort. It's about being there for them and providing reassurance.

The Connection between Mindful Speaking and Empathy:

Mindful speaking and empathy are closely intertwined because practicing mindful communication enhances your capacity for empathy:

Increased awareness: Mindful speaking encourages you to be more aware of your own thoughts and emotions, making it easier to connect with the emotions and perspectives of others.

Non-judgment: Mindful speaking's emphasis on non-judgment aligns with the non-judgmental approach of empathy, allowing you to listen without forming critical opinions about the other person.

Active listening: Mindful speaking involves active listening, a fundamental component of empathy, as it helps you truly understand the speaker's emotions and concerns.

Kindness and compassion: Both mindful speaking and empathy emphasize kindness, compassion, and respect, fostering a more empathetic and understanding communication style.

In conclusion, mindful speaking and empathy are complementary practices that enhance the quality of your interactions and relationships. By being fully present, self-aware, and compassionate in your communication, you can create a more empathetic and connected way of engaging with others, ultimately leading to improved understanding and stronger relationships.

Stress Management

Effective Stress Management is crucial for maintaining both mental and physical well-being. It involves adopting strategies and techniques to reduce and cope with the stressors that we encounter in our daily lives. Here are some of the key benefits of effective stress management:

Improved Mental Health: Managing stress can significantly reduce the risk of mental health problems such as anxiety and depression. Chronic stress can lead to the development or exacerbation of these conditions, so effective stress management can act as a preventive measure.

Enhanced Physical Health: Stress can take a toll on the body, contributing to various physical health issues, including heart disease, high blood pressure, and gastrointestinal problems. Stress management can help reduce the risk of these conditions and promote overall physical health.

Better Sleep: High stress levels can disrupt sleep patterns, leading to insomnia or poor-quality sleep. Stress management techniques, such as relaxation exercises and meditation, can help improve sleep quality and duration.

Enhanced Cognitive Function: Stress can impair cognitive function, making it difficult to concentrate, remember things, and make decisions. By managing stress, individuals can experience improved mental clarity and cognitive performance.

Increased Resilience: Learning how to effectively manage stress can enhance one's resilience, allowing them to better cope with life's challenges and bounce back from setbacks more easily.

Improved Relationships: Stress can strain relationships, as it can lead to irritability, mood swings, and decreased communication. Managing stress can help individuals maintain healthier relationships with family, friends, and colleagues.

Boosted Productivity: High stress levels can hinder productivity at work or in other areas of life. Effective stress management can help individuals stay focused and motivated, leading to increased productivity.

Enhanced Emotional Well-being: Managing stress can lead to greater emotional stability and a more positive outlook on life. It can help individuals experience more frequent positive emotions and a reduced frequency of negative ones.

Better Coping Skills: Stress management involves learning and practicing coping strategies, which can be applied not only to stress but also to other challenges in life. These skills can improve problem-solving abilities and emotional regulation.

Reduced Risk of Burnout: Chronic stress can contribute to burnout, which is characterized by emotional exhaustion, reduced performance, and a feeling of detachment from work or other responsibilities. Stress management can help prevent or alleviate burnout.

Enhanced Self-esteem: Successfully managing stress can boost self-confidence and self-esteem. As individuals gain control over their stressors, they often feel a greater sense of self-efficacy and self-worth.

Longer Life: Chronic stress has been linked to a shorter lifespan, mainly due to its negative impact on physical health. By effectively managing stress, individuals may increase their chances of living a longer, healthier life.

In conclusion, stress management offers a wide range of benefits that encompass both mental and physical well-being. By adopting various stress-reduction techniques and strategies, individuals can lead healthier, happier, and more fulfilling lives while minimizing the negative consequences of stress. It's important to note that different techniques work for different people, so it's essential to explore and find the stress management methods that suit your individual needs and preferences.

Meditation is a powerful tool for stress management and can

have a profound impact on your overall well-being. It offers a range of physical, mental, and emotional benefits that can help you cope with and reduce stress. Here's how meditation can assist with stress management:

Relaxation Response: Meditation triggers the relaxation response, which is the opposite of the body's stress response (fight-or-flight). When you meditate, your heart rate decreases, your breathing becomes slower and deeper, and your muscles relax. This counteracts the physical symptoms of stress.

Reduces Cortisol Levels: Cortisol is a hormone that's released in response to stress. Chronic stress can lead to elevated cortisol levels, which can have detrimental effects on the body. Meditation has been shown to reduce cortisol levels, helping to regulate the body's stress response.

Emotional Regulation: Meditation can improve emotional regulation, making it easier to manage stress-inducing emotions like anxiety and anger. By practicing mindfulness, individuals become more aware of their emotional reactions and better equipped to respond to them in a calm and measured way.

Improved Focus and Concentration: Stress can scatter your thoughts and make it difficult to concentrate. Meditation, particularly mindfulness meditation, can enhance your ability to focus by training your mind to stay in the present moment. This improved concentration can help you better manage the tasks causing you stress.

Enhanced Resilience: Regular meditation practice can build resilience to stress over time. It helps you develop a more balanced perspective on challenging situations, making it easier to bounce back from setbacks and adapt to change.

Better Sleep: Stress often leads to sleep disturbances. Meditation can improve the quality of your sleep by calming your mind and reducing racing thoughts, making it easier to fall asleep and stay asleep.

Lower Blood Pressure: High blood pressure is a common side effect of chronic stress. Meditation has been shown to help lower blood pressure, which is beneficial for overall cardiovascular health.

Reduced Muscle Tension: Stress can cause muscle tension, leading to discomfort and pain. Meditation can relax tense muscles, reducing physical symptoms of stress and promoting relaxation.

Enhanced Self-Awareness: Through meditation, you become more aware of your thoughts, emotions, and physical sensations. This self-awareness can help you identify stress triggers and implement proactive stress management strategies.

Mind-Body Connection: Meditation emphasizes the mind-body connection, fostering a holistic approach to well-being. It encourages you to pay attention to how stress affects your body and allows you to release tension and anxiety.

Increased Patience and Tolerance: Regular meditation practice can improve your patience and tolerance for frustrating situations, reducing the overall impact of stressors in your life.

To effectively harness the benefits of meditation for stress management, it's important to establish a consistent practice. Even just a few minutes of daily meditation can yield positive results over time. There are various meditation techniques to explore, such as mindfulness meditation, loving-kindness meditation, and transcendental meditation, so you can find the one that resonates with you the most. Additionally, combining meditation with other stress management techniques like exercise, a healthy diet, and social support can further enhance your ability to manage and reduce stress in your life.

———————————————

Creating a stress-resilient mindset

Creating a stress-resilient mindset involves developing psychological and emotional strategies to better cope with and bounce back from life's challenges and stressors. Here are some key steps to help you build a stress-resilient mindset:

Self-awareness: Start by recognizing your stress triggers and understanding how stress affects you physically and emotionally. Being aware of your stressors can help you prepare for them and develop strategies to manage them effectively.

Positive thinking: Cultivate a positive mindset by challenging negative thoughts and beliefs. Replace self-criticism and pessimism with self-compassion and optimism. Focus on your strengths and past successes to boost your confidence.

Mindfulness and meditation: Practicing mindfulness and meditation techniques can help you stay present in the moment and reduce the impact of stress. Regular mindfulness practice can improve your ability to respond to stressors calmly.

Healthy lifestyle: Prioritize physical health through regular exercise, a balanced diet, and adequate sleep. These factors play a crucial role in regulating stress hormones and promoting emotional well-being.

Time management: Develop effective time management skills to avoid feeling overwhelmed. Prioritize tasks, set realistic goals, and break large projects into smaller, manageable steps. This can reduce the pressure of deadlines and expectations.

Social support: Build a strong support network of friends, family, or colleagues. Sharing your thoughts and feelings with others can provide emotional relief and different perspectives on your problems.

Emotional intelligence: Enhance your emotional intelligence by understanding and managing your own emotions as well as the emotions of others. This skill can help you navigate stressful interpersonal situations more effectively.

Problem-solving skills: Develop your ability to identify problems, brainstorm solutions, and take action. A proactive approach to challenges can reduce stress by giving you a sense of control.

Resilience-building activities: Engage in activities that promote resilience, such as journaling, art, or creative expression. These activities can help you process emotions and develop a more resilient mindset.

Acceptance and adaptability: Understand that some stressors are beyond your control, and it's essential to adapt to changing circumstances. Embrace change as an opportunity for growth rather than as a threat.

Set boundaries: Establish clear boundaries in your personal and professional life. Saying "no" when necessary and prioritizing self-care can prevent burnout and excessive stress.

Seek professional help: If stress becomes overwhelming or chronic, consider consulting a therapist or counselor. They can provide valuable tools and strategies to manage stress and improve your resilience.

Celebrate successes: Acknowledge and celebrate your achievements, no matter how small they may seem. This can boost your self-esteem and provide motivation during challenging times.

Practice self-compassion: Be kind and compassionate toward yourself, especially when you make mistakes or face setbacks. Self-compassion helps you bounce back from difficult situations with greater resilience.

Learn from experiences: View challenging situations as opportunities for personal growth and learning. Reflect on past experiences to identify what you can do differently in the future.

Creating a stress-resilient mindset is an ongoing process that requires practice and self-reflection. By implementing these strategies and prioritizing your mental and emotional well-being, you can develop the resilience needed to navigate life's ups and downs more effectively.

Deepening Your Practice

Advanced breathing techniques

Advanced meditative breathing techniques go beyond basic mindfulness practices and involve more focused and deliberate control of your breath to achieve specific states of consciousness or deepen your meditation experience. These techniques require a foundation in mindfulness and meditation, so it's important to have some experience before attempting them. Always consult with a qualified meditation teacher or healthcare professional, especially if you have any pre-existing medical conditions.

Here are some advanced meditative breathing techniques:

Alternate Nostril Breathing (Nadi Shodhana): This technique involves using your thumb and ring finger to alternately close off one nostril while breathing in and out through the other. It's believed to balance the flow of energy in the body and calm the mind.

Box Breathing: In this technique, you inhale for a specific count (e.g., 4 seconds), hold your breath for the same count, exhale for the same count, and then hold your breath again. This pattern creates a square or box-like breath cycle and can help improve concentration and reduce anxiety.

Kapalabhati Breath: Kapalabhati is a forceful breathing technique in which you forcefully exhale through your nose while keeping your inhalations passive. It's thought to purify the body and mind by expelling stale air and toxins.

Sama Vritti (Equal Breathing): This technique involves inhaling and exhaling for an equal count, creating a balanced and rhythmic breath pattern. It can help calm the mind and improve focus.

Bhramari Pranayama (Bee Breath): Bhramari involves inhaling deeply and then making a low, buzzing sound like a bee while exhaling. It can help alleviate stress and anxiety and is often used as a precursor to meditation.

Ujjayi Breath: Ujjayi is characterized by a soft, ocean-like sound created by partially constricting the back of the throat while breathing in and out through the nose. It helps to enhance concentration and mindfulness during meditation.

Surya Bhedana and Chandra Bhedana: Surya Bhedana involves inhaling through the right nostril and exhaling through the left nostril, while Chandra Bhedana is the reverse, inhaling through the left nostril and exhaling through the right. These practices are believed to activate different energy channels in the body and influence your energy levels.

Kumbhaka (Breath Retention): Kumbhaka involves holding your breath after a deep inhalation or exhalation. It can be practiced with or without a specific pattern and is used to develop greater control over the breath and concentration.

Visualization with Breath: Combine deep, mindful breaths with visualization techniques. For example, you can imagine inhaling positive energy and exhaling negative energy or visualize your breath as a calming light that flows through your body.

Chakra Breathing: Focus your breath on specific energy centers or chakras in the body, imagining the breath entering and cleansing each one. This can help balance and align your energy centers.

Remember that advanced meditative breathing techniques should be practiced with caution and under the guidance of an experienced teacher. They can have powerful effects on the mind and body, so it's essential to approach them mindfully and with respect for your own limitations and comfort levels.

———————————————

Metta (Loving-Kindness) Meditation
Metta meditation, also known as Loving-Kindness med-

itation, is a Buddhist mindfulness practice that focuses on cultivating feelings of love, compassion, and goodwill towards oneself and others. The term "metta" is a Pali word, one of the languages used in early Buddhist texts, and it roughly translates to "loving-kindness" or "benevolence." Metta meditation is a popular form of meditation not only within Buddhism but also in secular mindfulness and contemplative practices.

Here is a step-by-step guide on how to practice Metta meditation:

Find a Quiet and Comfortable Space: Choose a quiet and peaceful place where you won't be disturbed. Sit or lie down in a comfortable position. You can close your eyes or keep them softly focused on a point in front of you.

Begin with Yourself: Start by directing metta (loving-kindness) towards yourself. Repeat a series of phrases or affirmations that express goodwill and kindness toward yourself. For example, you might say, "May I be happy. May I be healthy. May I live with ease."

Extend Metta to a Loved One: After a few minutes, shift your focus to a loved one—a family member, friend, or someone you deeply care about. Repeat the phrases, such as "May [their name] be happy. May [their name] be healthy. May [their name] live with ease."

Extend Metta to Neutral Individuals: Next, extend metta to neutral individuals—people you don't have strong feelings for one way or the other. It could be a neighbor, a coworker, or someone you encounter in your daily life.

Extend Metta to Challenging Individuals: This is often considered the most challenging part of Metta meditation. Send metta to someone with whom you have difficulties or conflicts. The goal is to foster understanding and compassion even in challenging relationships.

Extend Metta to All Beings: In the final stage, extend metta to all beings, without exception. You can use phrases like "May all beings be happy. May all beings be healthy. May all beings live with ease."

Conclude the Meditation: Gradually let go of the specific phrases and sit in a state of loving-kindness and openness for a few moments. Feel the sense of goodwill and warmth in your heart.

Return to Daily Life: When you are ready, open your eyes and carry the feelings of metta with you into your daily life, trying to interact with others in a more compassionate and loving way.

Metta meditation is not only a practice of self-care and self-compassion but also a powerful way to cultivate empathy, compassion, and a sense of interconnectedness with others. Regular practice can lead to increased feelings of kindness, reduced negativity, and improved relationships with both yourself and those around you.

Silent Retreats

Silent retreats offer a unique opportunity for individuals to disconnect from the noise and distractions of everyday life and immerse themselves in a peaceful and contemplative environment. These retreats typically involve a period of extended silence, often lasting several days or even weeks. While the experience can vary depending on the specific retreat and its focus (e.g., mindfulness, meditation, spiritual, or personal growth), there are several common benefits associated with silent retreats:

Deepened Inner Awareness: Silence allows participants to turn their attention inward, fostering a greater understanding of their thoughts, emotions, and inner processes. It can be a time for self-reflection and self-discovery, helping individuals gain insights into their lives and the choices they make.

Reduced Stress and Anxiety: The absence of external stimuli and the practice of mindfulness or meditation during silent retreats can significantly reduce stress and anxiety levels. This can have long-lasting effects on mental and emotional well-being, helping participants develop healthier coping mechanisms.

Improved Concentration and Focus: Continuous silence cultivates an environment where participants can concentrate deeply on the task at hand, whether it's meditation, self-reflection, or a particular practice. Over time, this enhanced focus can carry over into daily life, making it easier to stay present and attentive.

Enhanced Creativity: The absence of distractions can stimulate creativity. Many artists, writers, and thinkers have found silent retreats to be conducive to generating new ideas and gaining fresh perspectives on their creative projects.

Strengthened Relationships: Paradoxically, silent retreats can improve communication and relationships. By stepping away from the constant chatter and distractions of daily life, participants often gain a deeper understanding of themselves and others. This can lead to more meaningful and empathetic interactions when they return to the outside world.

Physical and Mental Health Benefits: The practice of mindfulness and meditation during silent retreats has been associated with various health benefits, such as lower blood pressure, improved sleep, and better pain management. Additionally, the reduction in stress and anxiety can positively impact overall mental and physical health.

Spiritual Growth: For those on a spiritual journey, silent retreats can provide a profound experience of connection, transcendence, and inner peace. They offer a chance to explore one's spiritual beliefs and practices in a focused and supportive environment.

Increased Mindfulness: Silent retreats often emphasize mindfulness practices, which can lead to greater awareness of the present moment and a deeper appreciation for life's small pleasures. This heightened mindfulness can help participants make more intentional choices in their daily lives.

Personal Growth and Transformation: Many people who attend silent retreats report experiencing personal growth and transformation. The extended period of silence and introspection can lead to profound shifts in perspective and a greater sense of purpose.

Digital Detox: Silent retreats typically involve a break from technology and the constant connectivity of the modern world. This digital detox can provide relief from information overload and the pressure to constantly be available, allowing participants to fully disconnect and recharge.

It's important to note that silent retreats can be challenging, especially for those unaccustomed to extended periods of silence and solitude. However, many participants find that the benefits far outweigh the initial discomfort, and they return from these retreats with a renewed sense of clarity, balance, and well-being.

The transformative power of nature sounds (or simple silence)

(For the purposes of meditation, we can spend time in a nature setting, far from the sounds of man-made hustle and noise, and still count that as "silence," even when birds are chirping and breezes blow.)

Even if you can't afford a silent retreat, something as simple as a road trip across town in a silent car, a half hour at an interstate scenic overlook, or a lunch break on the Appalachian Trail can be quite healing.

Silence has numerous benefits, both for our mental and physical well-being, as well as for our interpersonal relationships and overall quality of life. Here are some of the key advantages of embracing silence:

Stress Reduction:

Silence provides a break from the constant noise and stimulation of modern life, allowing the nervous system to relax and reduce stress levels. This can lead to lower blood pressure, reduced heart rate, and decreased cortisol levels.

Enhanced Focus and Concentration:

In a quiet environment, it's easier to concentrate on tasks, study, or work. Silence can help improve productivity and creativity by reducing distractions and allowing you to immerse yourself fully in what you're doing.

Improved Sleep Quality:

Noise pollution can disrupt sleep patterns, leading to sleep disturbances and insomnia. Creating a quiet sleep environment can result in more restful and restorative sleep.

Mindfulness and Meditation:

Silence is often associated with mindfulness and meditation practices. It allows individuals to become more in tune with their thoughts and feelings, promoting self-awareness and mental clarity. Regular meditation in silence can reduce anxiety and improve overall mental health.

Emotional Regulation:

Silence can provide a space for processing emotions and self-reflection. It allows you to disconnect from external distractions and connect with your inner self, facilitating emotional regulation and self-awareness.

Enhanced Communication:

In conversations and interpersonal relationships, silence can be a powerful tool. It allows for active listening and reflection, enabling more meaningful and thoughtful communication. Pauses in conversation can also convey empathy and understanding.

Creativity and Problem-Solving:

Silence can stimulate creativity and problem-solving by providing room for new ideas to emerge and for deeper thinking. It's during quiet moments that innovative solutions often come to mind.

Physical Health Benefits:

Studies have shown that chronic exposure to noise can have detrimental effects on physical health, including increased risk of cardiovascular diseases and cognitive decline. Embracing silence can help mitigate these risks.

Connection to Nature:

Spending time in natural settings where silence prevails can have a profound impact on well-being. Nature's silence allows for relaxation, rejuvenation, and a sense of connection to the environment.

Recharge and Self-Care:

Silence provides an opportunity to recharge mentally and emotionally. Engaging in moments of quiet reflection or simply enjoying a peaceful environment can be a form of self-care, promoting overall well-being.

Reduced Mental Fatigue:

Constant exposure to noise and information overload can lead to mental fatigue. Taking breaks in silence can help prevent cognitive overload and increase mental stamina.

Cultivation of Patience:

Silence can teach us patience by allowing us to become comfortable with the absence of constant stimulation. Learning to embrace quiet moments can lead to increased patience and tolerance in various aspects of life.

In a world filled with noise and distractions, incorporating moments of silence into our daily routine can have profound and positive effects on our physical and mental health, as well as our interpersonal relationships. It provides an opportunity to recharge, reflect, and reconnect with ourselves and the world around us.

Eight

Conclusion (for now...)

The Journey of Self-Discovery

The journey of self-discovery is a deeply personal and introspective process in which an individual seeks to gain a better understanding of themselves, their values, beliefs, emotions, desires, and purpose in life. It often involves reflecting on one's experiences, exploring one's inner thoughts and feelings, and evolving as a person. Here's an overview of the stages and key aspects of this transformative journey:

Self-awareness: The journey of self-discovery typically begins with self-awareness. This involves paying attention to your thoughts, emotions, and behaviors without judgment. It's about acknowledging your strengths, weaknesses, and patterns in your life. Journaling, meditation, and introspection are common tools for cultivating self-awareness.

Exploration of identity: As you become more self-aware, you'll start to question and explore your identity. This includes aspects such as your cultural background, values, beliefs, and personal interests. You may ask yourself questions like "Who am I?" and "What do I stand for?" This stage often involves a deep dive into your past experiences and upbringing to understand how they have shaped you.

Challenging assumptions: Part of self-discovery is questioning assumptions and beliefs that may not truly align with who you are or who you want to become. This can be a challenging process as it may involve letting go of long-held beliefs or reevaluating your priorities.

Emotional exploration: Understanding your emotions and how they influence your thoughts and behaviors is a crucial aspect of self-discovery. This involves recognizing and processing both positive and negative emotions, as well as learning healthier ways to cope with them.

Setting goals and values: As you gain a clearer understanding of yourself, you can start to define your core values and set personal goals that align with those values. This gives your life a sense of purpose and direction.

Facing fears and insecurities: Self-discovery often entails confronting fears, insecurities, and past traumas. It's about healing and finding ways to move forward. Therapy and counseling can be valuable resources during this stage.

Growth and self-improvement: Self-discovery is an ongoing journey of growth and self-improvement. It involves continuous learning, adapting, and evolving as a person. This may include acquiring new skills, expanding your knowledge, and working on personal development.

Self-acceptance: Ultimately, the journey of self-discovery leads to self-acceptance. This means embracing your true self, flaws and all, and being comfortable with who you are. It involves self-compassion and letting go of self-criticism and judgment.

Living authentically: Once you've discovered your true self and accepted it, you can start living authentically. This means making choices and decisions that are in alignment with your values and aspirations, rather than trying to conform to external expectations or societal norms.

Maintaining self-awareness: Self-discovery is an ongoing process. It's important to continue practicing self-awareness and periodically revisiting your values and goals to ensure they still resonate with who you are at any given stage in life.

The journey of self-discovery can be challenging and sometimes uncomfortable, but it can also be incredibly rewarding. It can lead to greater self-fulfillment, improved relationships, and a deeper sense of purpose in life. It's a continuous process that unfolds throughout one's lifetime, helping individuals become more authentic and more true to themselves.

————————

Reflecting on your meditation journey

Reflecting on your meditation journey can offer a range of valuable benefits that contribute to personal growth, mental well-being, and a deeper understanding of yourself and your practice. Here are some of the key advantages:

Increased Self-Awareness: Reflecting on your meditation journey encourages self-examination. It helps you become more aware of your thoughts, emotions, and behaviors both on and off the cushion. This self-awareness can lead to better self-understanding and personal growth.

Progress Tracking: Regular reflection allows you to track your progress in meditation. You can observe how your practice has evolved over time, noticing improvements in concentration, mindfulness, and the ability to handle stress or difficult emotions.

Identifying Patterns: Through reflection, you may start to notice recurring thought patterns or emotional triggers that arise during meditation. Recognizing these patterns can be the first step toward addressing and ultimately transcending them.

Deeper Insights: Reflection can lead to profound insights into your inner world. You may gain a deeper understanding of your motivations, desires, fears, and the root causes of your suffering. These insights can be transformative and lead to lasting changes in your life.

Stress Reduction: By reflecting on your meditation journey, you can identify specific techniques or approaches that are particularly effective at reducing stress and promoting relaxation. This allows you to tailor your practice to better suit your individual needs.

Enhanced Focus and Concentration: Over time, reflection can reveal how your ability to concentrate and focus has improved. Recognizing this progress can be motivating and encourage you to continue your meditation practice.

Emotional Regulation: Meditation often helps individuals regulate their emotions. Reflecting on your experiences can show you how meditation has influenced your emotional responses and helped you develop greater emotional resilience.

Better Decision-Making: As you become more aware of your thoughts and emotions, you may find it easier to make decisions with clarity and discernment. This can lead to better choices in various aspects of your life.

Improved Relationships: Meditation can also positively impact your relationships by making you more mindful and empathetic. Reflecting on your journey can highlight moments where meditation has helped you respond to others with greater kindness and understanding.

Motivation and Accountability: Regular reflection serves as a motivational tool. When you see the positive changes meditation brings to your life, you're more likely to stay committed to your practice and continue reaping its benefits.

Mindfulness Integration: Meditation is often about cultivating mindfulness, and reflection helps you integrate mindfulness into your daily life. It reminds you to be present, non-judgmental, and attentive to your experiences in every moment.

Resilience Building: Through reflection, you can recognize your growing resilience in the face of challenges. This awareness can bolster your confidence in dealing with life's difficulties.

Spiritual Growth: For those on a spiritual journey, meditation reflection can be a profound way to explore your inner spirituality, connect with a higher purpose, and deepen your sense of meaning and fulfillment.

Incorporating reflection into your meditation practice can be as simple as setting aside a few minutes after each session to journal your experiences, insights, and observations. Over time, this practice can enhance the overall benefits of meditation and support your personal development and well-being.

— — — — — — — — — —

Celebrating progress, no matter how small, is crucial for several reasons:

Motivation and Encouragement: Recognizing and celebrating small achievements can provide individuals with a sense of accomplishment and motivation. When people see that their efforts have yielded results, even if they are minor, they are more likely to stay committed to their goals and continue working towards them. This positive reinforcement can be a powerful force for sustained effort.

Positive Reinforcement: Celebrating progress reinforces the behavior that led to that progress. When you acknowledge and reward small wins, you are sending a signal to your brain that the actions you took were valuable and should be repeated. This positive feedback loop can help establish good habits and behaviors.

Building Confidence: Every success, no matter how small, contributes to building self-confidence. Confidence is a key driver of success, as it enables individuals to take on more significant challenges and believe in their ability to overcome obstacles. Celebrating small wins helps boost self-esteem and self-assurance.

Reduces Stress and Burnout: Pursuing long-term goals can be daunting and stressful. Celebrating small milestones along the way can provide relief from the pressure and stress associated with the journey. It breaks down a larger goal into more manageable pieces, making it feel less overwhelming.

Maintaining Perspective: Celebrating progress helps individuals maintain perspective on their journey. It's easy to get caught up in the end goal and become discouraged when it seems distant. Recognizing and celebrating small victories reminds individuals that they are making progress, even if they haven't reached their ultimate destination yet.

Fosters a Positive Environment: Celebrating progress isn't just beneficial for individuals; it can also create a positive and supportive environment in teams and organizations. When leaders and colleagues acknowledge and celebrate the achievements of team members, it promotes a culture of appreciation, collaboration, and camaraderie.

Adaptation and Learning: Celebrating small wins can also serve as an opportunity for reflection and learning. When you take the time to acknowledge what went right in achieving a small milestone, you can also assess what strategies worked and what can be improved. This reflective process contributes to personal and professional growth.

Long-Term Success: The journey towards any significant goal is often composed of a series of small steps. Neglecting to celebrate these steps can lead to burnout and demotivation. By celebrating progress along the way, individuals are more likely to persevere in the face of challenges and achieve long-term success.

In summary, celebrating progress, no matter how small, is not just a feel-good exercise; it plays a crucial role in motivation, confidence-building, stress reduction, and long-term success. It's a simple yet powerful tool that individuals and organizations can use to enhance their performance and well-being.

Encouragement and Final Thoughts

I never expected to overcome my tendency for mind-wandering as easily as I have, not that everyone can say the same. We all have our lives to live, on various paths that may or may not converge. Regardless of our circumstances we will always be able to reign in our thoughts to a certain degree – and when things get too big for the methods described here, we need to recognize that and deal with things before they get much bigger (and meditation can wait).

But the tough times do end, and recovery is the order of the day. We have used meditation previously to self-assess and prepare the proper growth plans, hopefully to make the tough times a bit smoother.

I can't tell you how many people I've met who haven't grown (from within) since High School. Very sad.

Please raise a virtual glass with me as I propose a toast: To Embracing Meditation as a Lifelong Practice. To removing any barriers to proper and healthy meditation, whether it be fear, or distractions, or thoughts of boredom. To the wonderful potential for lasting transformation!